SEEING RED

SEEING RED

The One Book Every Woman Needs to Read.
Period.

KIRSTEN KARCHMER

TILLER PRESS

New York   London   Toronto   Sydney   New Delhi

TILLER PRESS

An Imprint of Simon & Schuster, Inc.
1230 Avenue of the Americas
New York, NY 10020

First Tiller Press hardcover edition November 2019

TILLER PRESS and colophon are trademarks of Simon & Schuster, Inc.

For information about special discounts for bulk purchases,
please contact Simon & Schuster Special Sales at 1-866-506-1949
or business@simonandschuster.com.

The Simon & Schuster Speakers Bureau can bring authors to your live event. For more information or to book an event, contact the Simon & Schuster Speakers Bureau at 1-866-248-3049 or visit our website at www.simonspeakers.com.

Interior design by Davina Mock-Maniscalco

Manufactured in the United States of America

1   3   5   7   9   10   8   6   4   2

Library of Congress Cataloging-in-Publication Data has been applied for.

ISBN 978-1-9821-3195-1
ISBN 978-1-9821-3196-8 (ebook)

Medical Disclaimer

· · · · · · · · · ·

This publication contains the opinions and ideas of its author. It is intended to provide helpful and informative material on the subjects addressed in the publication. It is sold with the understanding that the author and publisher are not engaged in rendering medical, health, or any other kind of personal professional services in the book. The reader should consult his or her medical, health, or other competent professional before adopting any of the suggestions in this book or drawing inferences from it.

The author and publisher specifically disclaim all responsibility for any liability, loss, or risk, personal or otherwise, which is incurred as a consequence, directly or indirectly, of the use and application of any of the contents of this book.

For the ten thousand women who have trusted me with their hearts, minds, and bodies. You taught me how to decipher the beautiful and secret language of women's bodies.

Contents

· · · · · · · · · ·

Introduction

· · · · · · · · · ·

1.7 billion people on this planet menstruate.

That means that 4.2 million of them are having their periods right now.[1]

More than 80 percent of them suffer from significant and life-interrupting premenstrual syndrome and cramping.[2]

That is a really big deal for women and their health—so it's shocking that no one seems to be talking about it.

Until now.

If you are one of the 3.4 million women who are suffering every month, if your sister, friend, or daughter suffers, or if you're a partner of someone who is suffering, this book is for you.

Your menstrual cycle is a barometer of your health, and while I will teach you how to improve your period—and use your cycle as a diagnostic tool for your overall health—this book isn't really just a period fix-it book. It is an exploration of a world where women are filled with so much shame about their periods that they've suffered in silence for century after century. It is also about the impact it is having on both the quality of our lives and our access to power and freedom. Once you understand how this deeply rooted and systemic stigma affects us even today, I'll move on to helping you better understand your cycle and how to optimize it. Last, we look at what we, as menstruating people, can do as a community to liberate ourselves and others from the shame, stigma, and suffering of menstrual cycles so that we can reclaim our bodies, our health, and our identities and take over the world.

About Language

You will notice I shift back and forth between the terms *women* and *people with periods* (*PWPs*). This may seem unusual and even awkward, but I feel it's incredibly important to recognize that not every person who has a period identifies as a woman, and also that not every woman menstruates. Sometimes I will use the term *women* because I'm speaking of the struggles of those who historically have been identified as women, and situations unique to that group. But never do I intend to be exclusionary. I use the acronym PWPs frequently because I want this book to be part of a new vernacular of inclusivity, diversity, and acceptance.

About My Point of View

I was trained in both Western medicine and traditional Chinese medicine (TCM). I earned a master's degree in traditional Chinese medicine from the Academy of Oriental Medicine in Austin, Texas, where, alongside four years of coursework in acupuncture and herbal medicine, I also studied biochemistry, organic chemistry, reproductive physiology, and pathophysiology. I worked hand in hand with a reproductive endocrinologist developing and implementing strategies to optimize fertility outcomes. In fact, Reproductive Medical Associates (RMA) of Texas, a very well-known IVF center, had a clinic inside my Austin clinic. During my twenty-year clinical career working with women's reproductive health, I was fascinated by what real integrative medicine could look like in practice. I wanted to explore what happens when you combine the best of every clinical solution as a new system to significantly improve women's overall health instead of just focusing on one symptom with one intervention. Based on my experience, I developed my own version of integrative medicine that uses a diagnostic algorithm to combine a woman's symptoms, menstrual cycle characteristics, basal body temperatures, and habits to create customized interventions that allow me to get to the root of the problem and stop focusing on symptoms. This new paradigm borrowed from the best of many disciplines, like Western medicine, Chinese medicine, behavior science, nutrition, mind/body, and, ultimately, technology, and with it I realized that the way to improve any health problem is to diagnose and understand the relationship between all of the signs and symptoms and then attack them from every discipline. As you are reading, note that some of the ways I talk about physiological functions and methods of understanding the body may be different from conventional thinking and that they come from both my vast clinical experience and peer-reviewed data, so although they may be novel, they are not fabricated.

It is time for a paradigm shift around the thinking about women's health. How we are currently taking care of women and their health isn't working, so we have to be open to a new way of approaching our health in order to transcend a system that is disease and drug focused. Both of those elements play important roles in our medical system, but if 80 percent of women are sick each month, what we are doing needs a *huge* revision.

This book is the brainchild of the more than twenty years as a clinician in which I have had the distinct pleasure of improving the cycles and fertility of thousands of women. Whenever I tell women the kind of information I've included in this book, they almost always say the same thing:

Why doesn't every woman (or PWP) know this?

Now they can.

SEEING RED

1
....

WHAT THIS BOOK IS ABOUT AND WHY IT'S IMPORTANT

When I was a kid, I wanted *desperately* to grow up. My three sisters and brother were all almost ten years older than I, so I lived in a home populated predominantly by adults, and I wanted to be like them. When my mom was napping, I would sneak upstairs and play with my sisters' makeup, bras, and whatever else I could find that would make me feel connected to them. Their grown-up teenage world seemed mysterious and foreign to me, but I thought that if I could learn about it, I'd be able to join them. It never worked out well. I'd be in a trance rifling through their big basket of eye shadows, wearing my sister's bra with the DD cups over my dress, and humming "You're a rich girl, and you've gone too far . . . it's a bitch, girl, and you've gone too far" (swearing made me feel older, too, and I haven't outgrown that habit, as you'll soon learn). They'd usually catch me in the act and promptly lay into me for messing around with their stuff.

Back then, it had never even occurred to me that part of "growing up" meant getting your period. Despite the fact that I shared a house with four (count them!) menstruating women, I knew *very* little about the whole thing—until I was thirteen. It finally happened. I found blood in my underwear, showed my mom, and she promptly handed me a box of tampons. *Super* tampons! Yes, I said super. We were a very practical family, and I suppose that was all we had on hand. I doubt that it even occurred to my mom that a super tampon was probably *way* too big for a girl's first experience with so-called feminine protection. But you know what they say: what doesn't kill you makes you stronger!

Feeling *very* uncertain about what to do with the pink box in my hand (hell, I didn't even know what the heck a tampon was, much less where to put it to stop the bleeding), I decided to go to my bathroom—I liked to call it my office—to do some research. That "bathroom research" probably marked the beginning of my career-long study of women's health. Hiding securely behind my office's locked door, I opened the box and looked at those pink soldiers all packed together like sardines. I pulled one out, and I remember thinking how irritating it was that the tampon was swathed in all that plastic because it was going to make it very difficult to open and examine one of the fuckers without everyone in the whole house hearing that noisy crinkling sound. Nevertheless, I proceeded and found a neatly folded instruction sheet at the bottom of the box (like the prize at the bottom of a Cracker Jack box, except that the prize actually sucked).

When I opened the pamphlet, I was dumbstruck. I had no idea what I was looking at. Hell, I couldn't even figure out which end was up! It was like an Ikea diagram full of weird angles and language that was totally foreign to me.

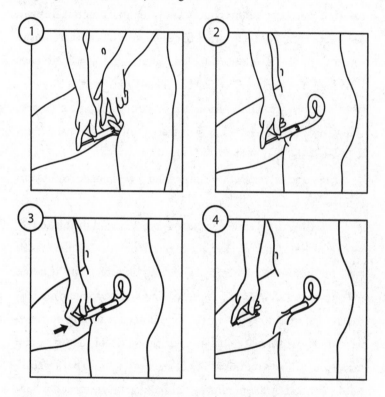

I wasn't completely unaware that women had periods, and I knew my mom and sisters had them (hence the supersize tampon box). But I just couldn't work up the nerve to ask them for help. Finally, I called my friends to help me figure it out. I had all of those women in my own home who could have easily guided me in the right direction, but I was too ashamed and embarrassed to ask. I grew up in a very close-knit family, but still I had absorbed the cultural norm that menstruation was something to hide.

Between the ages of thirteen and eighteen, I spent a ton of time doing gymnastics in a sweltering gym and thousands of hours on hot Texas tennis courts. I grew up in Arlington, Texas, a town renowned for being a city of cul-de-sacs where there wasn't much to do. I stayed out of trouble by training. I trained *really* hard four, five, six hours a day. I often kept going until I threw up from heat or exhaustion—or both. Of course, no one ever said, "Hey, that doesn't seem okay!" Instead, they said, "What a hard-working baller that girl is!"

Then one day, something happened that changed my life forever.

There I was, seventeen years old, practicing in the blistering, hot Texas sun. The court surface temperature was 117 degrees F., and the bottom of my feet were getting blistered right through my sneakers. I didn't care, though—I was so happy playing tennis. As I started to warm up (as if you need warming up when it's that hot), I threw the ball up, went to hit it for the serve, and the racquet flew right out of my hand. I thought, "That's weird," but I reasoned that sometimes your hand gets sweaty and it happens. Plus, I didn't want my super expensive new graphite racket to shatter, so I was worried that I hadn't been careful enough. So, I threw the ball up to serve a second time, and the racquet flew right out of my hand *again* and slammed down on the court. Then came the sinking feeling in my stomach. I'd always had a powerful serve, but there just didn't seem to be any strength in my hand to hold on to the racquet. I threw the ball up a third time. Want to take a guess on what happened next? The racquet flew out of my hand once again, and I knew that something was really, really super wrong. My whole right side was weak, and I had no grip strength; I just couldn't hold on to the damn racquet.

I didn't tell anybody. I put my racquet into the trunk of my car, drove away, and stopped playing tennis altogether. The tennis season was over, and surprisingly my parents didn't notice— maybe I lied and told them I was playing when I was really hanging out with friends, avoiding thinking about how weird my hand and the top of my leg felt. You couldn't tell by looking at me that anything was wrong, but I knew for sure. Tennis had been such a major part of my life, yet I went off to college knowing that something drastic had changed that I wasn't willing to face.

It wasn't just the weakness that signaled to me that I was sick; I was exhausted, and I was sleeping all the time. I had diarrhea six times a day. But I had been strictly trained as an athlete to ignore any sickness or sign of weakness. My father, who thought of me as his superstar kid, continually told me to "toughen up." And the fact that I'd stopped menstruating? I could completely ignore that—it wasn't a red flag, it was a badge of honor. But that day on the court was the first time I had to admit to myself that something was happening to me that I couldn't fix alone—and it only got worse. I became more and more tired. I noticed that when I was running, I wasn't getting the same sensation from the ball and toes of my right foot as I was from my left. I could still feel the pavement, but not in the same way. The weakness and exhaustion progressed faster and faster. I was ignoring all of the signals that something was seriously wrong, and this was a terrible idea that I do not endorse.

Enrolled at the University of Texas at Austin, I was a college student, finally all grown up. But I was still afraid to tell my family what was going on, thinking they would tell me, "Don't be a baby," or my father would say, "It's all in your mind." After all, I wasn't conventionally sick. But then I started to have trouble walking, and that was the one thing I just couldn't shake off—not being able to *walk*. I started using a cane because I was falling so much. Finally, I went to the UT health center. I saw a regular doctor, then a neurologist, as they tried to figure out what was happening with me. Even then, I still got a lot of "There's nothing wrong with you, it's just your imagination." But what became obvious over the course of that year was that my legs were less and less able to carry me. And I couldn't ignore that. After a lot of tests, including an MRI, I was diagnosed with multiple sclerosis at twenty years old. The thing about MS is that it has to reach a certain threshold before it can be diagnosed. I was ignoring it because my doctors kept telling me nothing was wrong; now I couldn't anymore—something was clearly wrong.

You might think this is crazy, but after all that, once I was finally diagnosed, I decided against the conventional drug treatments my doctors were proposing. At the time, there were no ten-year-plus studies on the drugs they wanted to give me. I didn't want to be a guinea pig for a new drug only to find out later it had some rotten side effects—like when women were given thalidomide for morning sickness, only to learn later that it had caused their children to have serious congenital deformities.

I didn't really have any other solutions to my problems, but a new, untested (at least for the long haul) drug wasn't going to be my first route. Unfortunately, MS is kind of episodic. Each time it flares up, it presents in a different way, so I never knew what to expect, what I was going to wake up to each morning. It was terrifying to know that I might wake up blind one day. But I've always trusted my gut, and my gut said, "No drugs, no treatment." That didn't mean I didn't want to get better. I just wanted to get better in a different way.

I had never let anything get in the way of what I wanted before, and I knew I wanted to travel. Even though I'd been given that diagnosis, I'd accepted a job in South Korea teaching English. Despite the fact that I was using a cane to walk at the time, I wanted to be able to explore other countries freely and not feel like a disabled person. I wanted to feel safe. So, I decided to start doing the Korean Special Forces Training, otherwise known as Tukong Moosul, or TKMS. TKMS emphasizes one or two quick, strategic strikes, after which you can run away (or hobble away, in my case) unscathed. A man can almost always overpower a woman in a longer fight, but this is just wham, bam, and outta there. It also incorporates using canes, so it was perfect for me. I got to use my disability as my weapon, so I could still kick ass!

•   •   •

Around that time, I had a lumbar puncture that left a tiny hole in my spinal cord. I was so depleted and exhausted that it wouldn't heal and was leaking cerebrospinal fluid (CSF) whenever I was upright. The longer I sat or stood, the more leaked out, and ultimately, I would pass out. Once I was lying down, my CSF returned to equilibrium and I'd be fine. I didn't really think it was a big deal. Mostly I considered it a giant pain in the ass. I even had a surgery called a blood patch to "plug the hole" that was unsuccessful as well.

Finally, though, one of my friends who was in acupuncture school said, "You should go to my teacher. I bet he could fix that." I didn't mention that I'd already had surgery to attempt to "fix the leak," but I did rebuff her; I thought having acupuncture was about as valid as going to a psychic—total bullshit. Eventually, I ended up going to see the acupuncturist, mostly to humor my friend. To make it fun, though, I refused to help that "psychic" con me, so I decided, "I won't tell him anything; I'll hide my cane and my chart, and let's just see what happens."

The first thing he did was take my pulse for a long time; then he asked me if I was "so tired." I thought, "Well, everybody's tired. He's just going for the low-hanging fruit." Then he asked, "You cannot digest food?" And that was really true; I still had loose stool six times a day. But I was sure a lot of people had digestive issues. Then he cocked his head and asked me if I had muscle weakness. Remember, he hadn't seen my chart, and he didn't know that I was using a cane. I hadn't said anything about muscle weakness, so how did he know? I said, "I have multiple sclerosis." He started clapping and saying, "I'm so happy, so happy!" Surprised, I asked, "*Why* are you so happy?" He said, "Because that makes perfect sense. Your body is so weak, there is no help to convert the food you are eating into energy. If you can't turn your food into energy, you cannot turn the energy into blood.

Without adequate blood, you cannot nourish the brain, muscles, and nervous system." I was dumbstruck. I thought, "He's actually right. That is so simple and obvious. Why doesn't everyone think this way about the body and medicine?"

That was a pivotal moment for me. That's when I turned the corner mentally and, eventually, physically. The acupuncturist helped me to understand that I had been born with multiple sclerosis but my constitution, or my base health, was incredibly strong, stronger than the disease. But then, because I was a little overachiever Energizer Bunny, training so many hours in the gym and playing tennis, sweating and throwing up every day, ultimately my body had become depleted and the disease had gotten stronger. When that happened, MS had presented itself, I had started showing symptoms, and had finally been diagnosed. The acupuncturist believed that we could make my constitution stronger than the disease, and if we could do that, it would go into remission.

Imagine the light bulb going off over my head with a little *hallelujah* on the side!

Everything he'd said felt right to me: Your ability to make blood and regulate it all goes back to your ability to break down food and turn it into energy. An autoimmune disease is like having a bunch of uncontrolled kids racing around your house and writing on your walls with Sharpies—it's your body crying out. It takes a robust constitution to manage the immune system—to get those kids to sit down and play nice.

That is when I decided to study acupuncture and started looking at schools that could train me. I needed to know more. All

I could think about was my hunger for knowledge about a world of medicine that was so new and inspiring to me. I was about to set off for Korea, but I figured that I could study Chinese medicine there, near the source. But you know what? I didn't really get the chance, because it wasn't in vogue! Anytime I got sick while I was there and asked for an acupuncturist, my Korean friends laughed at me and said, "That's only for grandparents. We'll take you to the new hospital." Even the acupuncturist I *did* visit in Korea asked me, "What are you doing here? Most young people go to the hospital." I was, as I would be so many times in my life, the anomaly.

Before acupuncture, I'd have MS episodes, and my symptoms (anything from sheer exhaustion to a droopy eye) would remain for three to four months and then slowly get better. But within the first ninety days of my weekly acupuncture treatment, the episodes started happening less frequently and getting better faster. I've been symptom free for twenty-five years now. It helps that I can treat myself if I need to, but I've also learned to listen to my body's signals. I have to pay attention all the time. I meditate every day. I try to watch what I eat. Though I don't have to eat *perfectly* every day, I try to be sure I'm getting enough nutrients (as getting energy from food is not one of my body's strong points). Insomnia is my biggest issue, so I don't have the stamina to work eight hours straight. I take a nap around two, and then I'm good again. But you know, crazy as it sounds, being diagnosed with MS was really the best fucking thing that's ever happened in my life. I learned what it means to be a very sick person, how to be around people who are also sick, and how much effort it takes to transcend the health issues you've been stuck in for what seems like forever.

• • •

As I was studying acupuncture—later specializing in reproductive acupuncture—I realized that understanding a patient's menstrual cycle enriched my ability to construct a really good diagnosis. Every aspect of the cycle tells you so much, giving you the ability to use it as a very precise diagnostic tool. In Chinese medicine, it's not the chicken or the egg, it's the chicken *and* the egg—things happen simultaneously. Nothing's separate in the body; just as my first acupuncturist proved to me with MS, everything is connected.

Now, if you think about the body from a Western medical perspective, you might be thinking, "No, MS is an autoimmune disease. Either you have it or you don't." And that there is no data to support a causal link between digestion and MS. But if you think about it, your body can make resources for well-being and healing only if it's able to take in food, break it down, and convert it into energy effectively. Typically, we think about digestion as elimination, aka pooping, but the function of digestion is determined by the Krebs cycle and our ability to make ATP (energy), possibly the earliest aspects of cellular metabolism to evolve. The Krebs cycle is a series of chemical reactions used by all aerobic organisms to make energy. That is the biochemical aspect of digestion, but from an Eastern and holistic point of view, it is the mechanism in which food becomes usable energy.

If this can't be done successfully, your disease will thrive and you'll continue to decline.

When I was really sick with MS, I didn't have a period. My poor digestion had left me with a "blood deficiency." Once I started getting better, I saw changes. My period started again and began to have more volume, and my muscles got stronger. The improvement was progressive, maybe 10 percent a month, and I hadn't yet tied the disease to my menstrual cycle. Only when I looked backward did I realize how important a diagnostic tool my cycle was. I saw it in my practice, too, after I graduated four years later.

Once I was in practice, I was seeing hundreds of fertility and reproductive patients a week and started to see some correlations between a woman's cycle and her overall health. These patterns were so strong and gave me so much information about the woman's overall health, that I got to the point where I was exclusively using the menstrual cycle as my primary diagnostic tool. I became so obsessed with the menstrual cycle that I didn't want to see men in my practice anymore because they didn't menstruate. The menstrual cycle not only gave me cues to make a really precise diagnosis but also provided a monthly feedback mechanism to measure success. I started thinking about Chinese medicine in a new way. Typically, the medical discipline is reactive: you identify the chief complaint and associated symptoms, feel the patient's pulse, look at the patient's tongue, and choose a treatment. It's simple: your diagnosis is based upon what you see that day; you are reacting to the current presentation. But I used the menstrual cycle to plan my attack ahead of time, before the symptoms hit—for the next four weeks, for a full month, I was *pro*active. I was looking at every sign and symptom, even the ones the patient wasn't currently experiencing, to create a precise picture of her entire ecosystem—and beyond that, diagnosing how all her signs, symptoms, and habits were related.

In 2000, I opened one of the first reproductive acupuncture clinics in the United States, where I took care of thousands of women with fertility and reproductive issues. I noticed that those who couldn't get pregnant had really bad periods and basal body temperatures that spiked up and plummeted down like EKG graphs. Typically, basal temperatures are used to predict ovulation and the date of your next period, but I started seeing patterns in the temperatures that allowed me to also use them diagnostically. As my patients' cycles and temperatures were regulated, they became healthier, and they were also significantly more likely to get pregnant. This system became so predictable that I started using the menstrual cycle and temperature patterns as the barometer of other health issues and the road map for correcting them. After seeing this literally thousands of times, I was able to really narrow down what the ideal cycle looks like. The "unicorn cycle"—I joke about that because women always tell me, "That's a unicorn"—has no pain whatsoever. There is no cramping, no clotting, no spotting. There are fresh red blood and biphasic temperatures, with the appropriate difference between the follicular phase (the first fourteen days of the cycle) and the luteal phase (second fourteen days). This cycle became my goal for all of my patients because I'd realized that even for women who aren't trying to get pregnant, the "unicorn cycle" represents optimal health.

The striking thing was that when I'd tell women about regulating their cycle and how it can be used as a diagnostic tool for fertility and overall health status, *they'd get mad*! Not at me but because they'd never heard anyone say anything like that before. They would often cry a bit and say something like "I'm thirty-eight years old, and I've been suffering for a long time. Why is this the first time anyone's ever told me this?"

I've always felt sick thinking about how so many women suffer needlessly. I don't have the power to fix most of the suffering on the planet, but I can fix menstrual suffering. I needed to do this.

• • •

Eventually I stopped calling myself an acupuncturist. Not because I don't love acupuncture but because what I was taking—okay, "borrowing"—from Chinese medicine went beyond sticking needles into people. My new system gave me the ability to diagnose a woman's total ecosystem from her signs and symptoms: menstrual cycle characteristics, basal temperatures, stress levels, how much she exercises or doesn't, how much sleep she's getting, and other lifestyle habits that affect long-term health, wellness, and disease. All of those things come together to give a clear picture of how well a person's system is functioning as a whole—and this systems-oriented approach is what allows for precise, actionable treatment. This ability to treat the whole system and then create highly customized, multidisciplinary interventions is hugely beneficial. What is *really* amazing is that you don't have to fix all the individual symptoms; you just have to be able to figure out how the problem areas are related and then determine the order of operations that will work best to resolve them. Figure out how each of these pieces are connected and combine that analysis with the best of other impactful disciplines, such as nutrition therapy, Western medicine, mind/body work, and stress management, and suddenly you have a powerful intersection: precision medicine meeting with behavioral change tools, which results in profound improvements in women's health.

This strategy was super effective, but I felt limited and frustrated knowing that even though my treatments were significantly cheaper than IVF, many women couldn't afford either. Many women couldn't afford to see me in my clinic, either. I didn't feel okay about leaving them out in the cold. So, I set out to see if I could translate the program I ran in my clinic to a tech-enabled platform in order to make the treatments virtually free.

The company that came out of that idea, Conceivable, was an effort to try to democratize access to fertility care. I knew that more women like the ones who had been to my practice were suffering: seven million in the United States alone. I wanted to teach all that I knew about my specific perspective on integrative medicine, so that all people with periods (PWPs) who had never met me could use it. My team and I ended up producing highly successful user-friendly app technology that was able to predict and significantly increase the likelihood of natural conception. We taught this technology to collect the normal data you would gather with garden-variety period trackers, but instead of just predicting when you are going to ovulate or when you'll start your period, it could go through the whole diagnostic process I would do with a patient in person. The algorithm could then figure out how to address the problems based on the person's cycle metrics, her regular signs and symptoms, and the habits that contribute to them. It can actually give the user prescriptive tools to not only fix her symptoms but also change her whole health ecosystem.

As we were launching Conceivable, I was writing for a bunch of publications about periods and fertility. I wrote one article in particular for *Goop* magazine entitled "What Your Period Can Tell You About Your Health." That article resulted in hundreds of email responses saying, "Look, I'm twenty-six years old. I'm not even in a relationship. I don't want to have a baby right now. In fact, I'm not touching anything called Conceivable, but I heard you know how to fix periods. Do you think you could help me? I'm really suffering every single month."

I suddenly realized that there were many more than the 7 million women who couldn't get pregnant who needed my help (more like 82 million in the United States alone), and if I shared the strategies, products, and technologies that I developed, ultimately, I might be able to help more women prevent infertility and future disease. Creating resources for women even before they started their periods and continuing through menopause would enable me to support and educate women all across the reproductive life cycle. More than 80 percent of all women of menstruating age in the United States experience significant, life-interrupting side effects from their periods every month. In addition to addressing fertility issues, we could start to really reduce the impact and incidence of cramping as well as more serious underlying conditions such as polycystic ovarian syndrome (PCOS), endometriosis, recurrent pregnancy loss, and the struggles women have with menopause. We could stop acting as though all this is normal, because it is not. These numbers of women with menstrual disease represent epidemic conditions, and many of these conditions are highly correlated with the diseases that kill women (heart disease, type 2 diabetes, stroke, and estrogen-dependent tumors) every day.[1]

That was when I got really excited. I decided that that was the work to which I would devote myself for the rest of my life.

• • •

Yes, times are changing; women are marching and calling out "Time's up." But how can we possibly take our place, defend our rights, and demand equality when most of us are sick from our periods every month?

If our goal as a society is to really empower women, we have to start with women's health. A woman's cycle is not a curse but possibly the most valuable, regularly occurring, and free feedback tool a woman can use to measure her overall health. It can also provide a road map for fixing it and improving her current and future health, as well as quality of life, and access to power, and freedom. That's my goal for this book—part manifesto and part practical, data-driven guide to optimal health and wellness through understanding and embracing your period.

It's time we broke the silence surrounding the messy, uncomfortable matters related to the female body. It's time we started SEEING RED.

2
· · · · · · · · ·

THE HISTORY OF THE PERIOD

Nothing Has Changed for
Menstruating Women in Centuries

Those who cannot remember the past are condemned to repeat it.
—GEORGE SANTAYANA

When I was building my second company, Brazen, I read all of the epidemiologic literature about what I call "menstrual disease." These are all of the significant symptoms and diseases that affect women throughout the life of their reproductive cycle. Even though I had been fixing periods for well over twenty years, I'd never looked at the pervasiveness of menstrual disease. I never realized how many women suffered in some way every month from their periods and that most of them thought it was normal. I'd always been looking at it as a factor of infertility—not as a massive problem in its own right.

I knew that about one in seven women were infertile, but

I was shocked, dumbfounded, and speechless when I read that 82 percent of women, or about 75 million, in the United States alone reported that they had significant premenstrual syndrome (PMS) and cramping every month. I kept asking myself "How can we be in the middle of a women's movement with the majority of us still so sick—and *no one is talking about it*?" Worse, no one was doing anything about it.

I wanted to figure out why it seemed okay for so many women to suffer every month and for pretty much everyone to think that it wasn't a problem—even the women themselves! Being a former cultural linguist, I started my exploration by looking at how the history of language has played a role in our present-day lack of communication about women's periods and the illnesses related to them. I decided to go back to the beginning of written history to explore the way society has talked and related to women—and their periods.

What I found astounded me. I discovered that many cultures have systematically conditioned women to believe that our cycles are a kind of sickness that makes us feeble and inferior or unclean. It was extremely common in earlier times to perpetuate the myth that women are "limited" by having periods—or, worse yet, they'd be sequestered away from the rest of society while they were bleeding. Only on rare occasions since the beginning of written history have we taken the initiative to teach women that our cycles are simply a part of being a woman; suffering *because* of them doesn't have to be.

The History of Menstruation,
or the Lack Thereof

As I researched, I realized what was more important than what was written about women and their periods was what was *not* written.

Despite the fact that women have been menstruating since the beginning of human evolution, there is very little documentation about women's periods in ancient times. For the first 1,500 years of written language, I couldn't find one reference to menstruation except in Chinese medicine texts. Apart from that there was relative radio silence. It's as if menstruation didn't exist, even in medical and religious texts—probably in part because men were the only people who were taught to write but more likely because menstruation was considered such a taboo subject (the term *taboo* comes from the Tongan *tapu* and is used to signify something excessively repulsive or too sacred for ordinary folk— anything forbidden or restricted, such as incest, patricide, or cannibalism).

Earlier civilizations, from Mesopotamia to Greece, despite their many differences, all shared the same approach to describing women's periods: silence. Spanning more than half a dozen diverse cultures, almost no society that left written records mentioned the subject. The only culture that was talking about it were the scholars of traditional Chinese medicine around the year 200 BCE.

I don't know about you, but I find this incredible—and really disturbing.

From what we can see—even from the silence—period prejudice goes way back. Of course, we really don't know what women thought about their periods, because the men were doing the majority of the writing. But no matter where and when they're from, as texts began to occasionally mention the menstrual cycle, the message from most sources was that women who are menstruating are filthy and should be avoided until they are cleansed of their (and I'm not exaggerating here) "pollution."

The first widely public statements about menstruation come from the book of Leviticus in the Bible around the year 500 BCE. Whoever wrote it was a big fan of menstruating women and couldn't wait to get near some ladies on the rag. Kidding. The book perceives menstruating women as filthy and, quite frankly, dangerous to a man's soul. It says:

> Whenever a woman has her menstrual period, she will be ceremonially unclean for seven days. Anyone who touches her during that time will be unclean until evening. Anything on which the woman lies or sits during the time of her period will be unclean. . . . If a man has sexual intercourse with her and her blood touches him, her menstrual impurity will be transmitted to him. He will remain unclean for seven days, and any bed on which he lies will be unclean. . . . When the woman's bleeding stops, she must count off seven days. Then she will be ceremonially clean. On the eighth day she must bring two turtledoves or two young pigeons and present them to the priest at the entrance of the Tabernacle.[1]

Similarly, the Quran (2.222) has this to say about menstruating women: *"It is an impurity, so keep away from women during it and do not approach them until they are cleansed; when they are cleansed you may approach them as God has ordained."*[2]

If you are a Shinto, one of the main religions in Japan, menstruating women are not only impure during their cycle—they are permanently impure solely due to the fact that they menstruate. Not only are they forbidden to enter shrines due to their impurity, they're also forbidden to climb certain "sacred" mountains due to, you guessed it, that same "impurity."[3] I feel the urge to say, "Oh, come on . . ."

Then in the thirteenth century, someone you've probably heard of, Saint Thomas Aquinas, described a woman as a "misbegotten male." He wrote, *"The woman is defective and misbegotten for the active power in the male seed tends to the production of the perfect likeness according to the masculine sex; while the production of a woman comes from the defect in active power or from some material in this position or from some material indisposition, or from external influences, such as that of a south wind which is moist."* The inferiority of women is explained as the result of her menstrual flow, believed to be passive and "moist," therefore imperfect as an agent of procreation.[4]

This way of thinking has been pervasive up through the centuries until, well, pretty much now, as we'll get into later. So, we had the trusted and revered church—practically any church—telling us that we were both physically and spiritually filthy. As for science, well, Thomas was in total agreement with the third-century BCE words of one of the greatest thinkers of all time, Aristotle, who long before him had said the following:

> The outward sign of the female inferiority is menstruation. The female is deficient. Women are the inferior species . . . because they menstruate. They only contribute the serum [blood] in which the seed [sperm] can grow. The serum contributes the nutrition but the seed is the source of the spirit and intellect.[5]

And did science progress? Not so much. Even in 1878, letters to *The British Medical Journal* claimed that menstruating women would cause bacon to putrefy, and in 1916, the registrar of the Royal College of Physicians, Sir Raymond Crawford, wrote that farmers still believed that menstruating women would prevent milk from turning to butter or hams from curing.[6]

These falsehoods were the prevailing medical thought about women and menstruation even into the twentieth century! Yes, that is *centuries of conditioning*.

As I was discovering that, I kept wondering "Why is no one talking about this age-old attitude? Why have we just accepted this idea that our periods are a curse to be endured, that we are filthy and inferior because we menstruate?" Certainly, these conversations were going on in feminist scholarly circles, but they appeared to be absent in the conversations women were having with their colleagues and friends.

For centuries, women have experienced systematic conditioning (a nicer way of saying brainwashing), which has created an environment in which monthly menstrual suffering is accepted. Please notice, I do not use the word *victim*, because I don't want anyone to be a victim of anyone or anything. Looking through the lens of victimhood would disempower us from moving away from what's happened in the past into what we design for the future. But let's admit that this has not been an empowering situation for us—at least until now.

My question has been, But why have we put up with this? I'm pretty sure that men would never accept the shaming or the suffering. Not because they're smarter, better, stronger, or any of that patriarchal bullshit. But because they don't believe they have to. Of course, this belief derives from privilege, which drives an entirely different set of pathological behaviors—think #timesup, right? Still, it's useful to explore what men might do if they were in the same situation.

I have a little fantasy of attaching menstrual cramp simulators to men's balls for a day to see what would happen. Think about it: If I went into Congress tomorrow, attached those cramp-inducing mini machines onto the male congresspeople's balls, passed out cupcakes, bottles of Tylenol, and boxed wine, told them, "I'll be back in the morning!" and then left them to suffer through the night with the toolbox most of us use to manage a bad night of period cramps, what do you think would happen?

I think by the next morning, they'd all be saying "That shit is *never* happening again!" They would find a way to shut the country down and order the world's most brilliant experts on periods to solve the problem before their next cycle.

But women continue to suffer in silence.

I'm no psychologist, but I have a sense that our acceptance started with all those early conversations that influenced our self-worth at the deepest place. I think we internalized some part of that story as the truth.

I recently spoke with a very high-profile woman who is originally from India. She's a very forward-thinking medical doctor here. She shared a story about when her father died a few years ago. She went back to India for his funeral and got her period as soon as she arrived in her hometown. That created a real dilemma for her, because menstruating women are not allowed in the temples—even for their own father's funeral. She really didn't know what to do, because she doesn't consider herself a Hindu anymore and no one else would have known that she was menstruating, but still some part of her felt tremendous guilt about going against the religious proscriptions.

I'm not going to tell you what she decided in the end, because what I want to point out instead is that so many of us face this kind of choice. Even when we think we know better, that we've freed ourselves from these constricting ideas, we still face choices in our everyday lives that are impacted by them. We discover that even when we think, "Shit, there's no way I feel any menstrual shame"—whether it's feeling shy about having sex during our periods or hating to buy tampons from the teenage clerk at the drugstore—we do. The stories we're exposed to about our maturation, our bodies, our periods, and our fertility penetrate powerfully into our mind-set and can drive our thoughts and actions for our entire lives.

Managing Menstrual Blood
Through the Centuries

We can't look at the history of menstruation without examining how women and PWPs have managed their menstrual blood—especially when it was considered more vile than the Devil, which made it infinitely more important to hide any telltale signs.

Since we started with Leviticus above, let's first look at the prescriptions from the Bible. The Bible defines time frames for how long women are unclean after their periods—and how long anyone who touches them is unclean.[7] The Egyptians helped sanitize periods with the first tampons—too bad they were made out of papyrus—yes, rolled paper. Yikes, I can't imagine how uncomfortable those puppies were. If I'd been around back then, the entrepreneur in me would have been brainstorming like crazy how to improve the user experience and figure out a better material!

Now, to be fair, they did soften the papyrus in the Nile, but unfortunately, that's where most of the real "pollution" existed—given it was where most people bathed, washed their clothes and dishes, and probably used the bathroom at the time—so it couldn't have been healthy for women. At least they were reusable if you could find clean water to wash them. I can't believe that all menstruating women didn't die from the first cases of toxic shock syndrome![8]

Women in Victorian England decided that the plug-type solution was for the birds and just started free bleeding into their clothes—as late as the nineteenth century. I guess if your dress is poofy enough, you can hide any amount of blood underneath. I find that harder to wrap my mind around than even a papyrus tampon.[9]

During World War I, French nurses got the great idea of making pads out of wood pulp bandages. At last! I'm not sure why it took so long for the whole world to figure that one out. Despite the fact that those first pads were pretty big and cumbersome, the idea took off all over the world thanks to those trendsetting Frenchwomen.[10]

By the 1920s, a lot was changing for women and their periods. Though pads did a great job of absorbing menstrual flow, they were traps for fecal and urinary bacteria (which in many ways they still are, and some nonorganic ones are chock full of dioxin). Women were dissatisfied with the ability of pads to keep them feeling fresh, which was probably the impetus for the first tampon as we know it. Invented by a doctor of osteopathic medicine, Earle Haas, the first tampon was originally known as the "catamenal device."[11] I can only assume he named it that after the Greek word for menses, but he doesn't seem to have explained his reasoning at the time for developing such an obscure term for something we PWPs use on a regular basis. However, we do know that he got the idea from a woman friend who had started simply inserting a piece of sponge inside herself, rather than wearing it outside. That made really good sense to the doctor, because physicians had already been using cotton to stop bleeding internally and externally. If the cotton were compressed, he apparently realized, it might be able to deliver longer-lasting absorbency.

Though the catamenal quickly grew in popularity, it took

a woman to really bring it to life. In 1936, a Denver business-woman, Gertrude Tendrich, bought Haas's company and re-named it Tampax. The rest is tampon history.[12]

*   *   *

Unfortunately, around the same time, there was a pretty serious setback in our journey to menstrual acceptance and freedom, thanks to Béla Schick, a pediatrician most famous for the "Schick test" used to detect exposure to diphtheria toxin. Evidently, one afternoon, he received a bouquet of ten dark red roses, which a maid placed in a vase of water. When he saw the next morning that the flowers had wilted and died, he made inquiries and discovered that the maid had been menstruating. The maid reported that often when she touched flowers during her period, they would die by the next day.

Seeing an opportunity to do some serious medical research, Schick then carried out experiments with menstruating and non-menstruating servant girls, checking the effect their status had on flowers and also on making dough. He concluded that something was excreted through the skin of menstruating women that had a toxic effect—very powerful toxins that he called *menotoxins*—creative, eh?[13, 14]

Schick thought menotoxins were some pretty nasty toxins present in menstrual blood right before and during the first few days of the onset of a woman's period. His and other "research" concluded that menotoxins had an inhibitory effect on the growth of roots, stems, bread dough, and seedlings. Menotoxins were still being discussed almost fifty years later in *The Lancet*, a major medical journal—meaning that some doctors were still giving that bogus theory real scientific credit in the 1970s![15]

Even as companies today such as Thinx and DivaCup are starting to change the conversation around menstruation, we're still deeply impacted and influenced by the mostly male-led corporations manufacturing menstrual products, marketing teams created by male ad executives, and religious leaders who tell us how to feel about our periods and bodies. As recently as 1997, advertisements for drugs meant for menstrual pain used the term *hygienic crisis*. Advertising has tremendous power to influence the tone of and attitudes in the cultural zeitgeist. Given that the entire messaging around menstrual products has been centered around "hygiene," it's quite clear how these very old belief systems have remained in place. But don't just believe me. Head over to your local Target, walk down the tampon aisle, and see just how many vaginal douches (extremely bad for your vaginal health), scented tampons, and vaginal fragrance sprays are available. Hell, the aisle is called "Feminine Hygiene"—merchandising in the name of sanitizing our crotches. I wish there was a row in the men's underwear aisle called "Skidmark Central"—then I might feel less discriminated against.

I'm guessing that most of this history is news to you. Again, that goes back to the fact that nobody talks about periods. What's especially galling—if not downright evil—is how we, as women, are supposed to make sure it stays that way. As Chris Bobel, the president of the Society for Menstrual Cycle Research and an associate professor of women's, gender, and sexuality studies at the University of Massachusetts, puts it, "The message to women has been: 'Menstruation is your problem, ladies. Your job is to render it invisible.'"[16] After speaking with thousands of women about their periods, I would say that most of us agree with that assessment. Even today, this attitude permeates almost every mainstream advertisement about menstrual products (which, paradoxically, are one of the few sources we *do* have for "information"), which always include the recurring themes of secrecy and the need for sanitization.

So where does that leave us?

Well, in 1981, Tampax, Inc., published a study called "The Tampax Report," which found that attitudes about periods and the people who have them are pretty dismal. Though this study is almost forty years old, according to Procter & Gamble (which now owns Tampax) the findings are still right on the money. Here is what the researchers found:

- One-third of American women were not prepared for menstruation, and two-fifths report their first reaction to it to have been a negative one.

- One-quarter of Americans think women cannot function normally at work while menstruating.

- One-half the population thinks that women should not have sexual intercourse while menstruating.

- One-third believe that menstruation affects a woman's thinking ability.

- One-third think women should restrict their physical activity during menstruation.

- Nearly one-quarter think that menstrual pain is all in a woman's head.

Other noteworthy findings focused on the differences between men and women's views on menstruation:

- 56 percent of women say menstruation is painful, but only 39 percent of men believe that.

- 88 percent of women and 66 percent of men think menstruation has no effect on work life.

- 38 percent of men and only 27 percent of women believe it's okay to talk about menstruation.

So we still have some work to do. But we can get there.

Taking Back the Power

Here's what I find incredibly ironic: women have been shamed, subjugated, mutilated, beaten, and cast out because they bled. We have been demeaned and labeled by the Church and scientific leaders as filthy, feeble, and inferior. But in reality, folks are super fucking scared of the mysterious power of menstrual blood. Unfortunately for women, it's fairly easy to indoctrinate the young, ripe minds of adolescents into the dominant belief system—and they may never break free of those ideas.

Historically, when young women first get their periods, many cultures have directly or indirectly let them understand exactly how their community feels about them and their maturing, menstruating bodies. From forced seclusion and beating to cutting and circumcising, the rituals that are performed when a young girl starts her period send a clear message that now that you're a woman, you need to be docile and agreeable.

The question is, Why is that so important? The majority of taboos and myths around menstruation stem from the fear that menstruating women's power to also create signals they have the power to destroy, and that power must be contained for the well-being of society—or, maybe just the well-being of men in order to enforce their economic power in society. Just sayin'.

Fear and the desire for power or control drive almost everything in our society, and it's easy to see how rituals, taboos, and mythology have set the tone around menstruation since practically the beginning of time. Let's look at just a few examples of the mighty power of menstrual blood that illustrate exactly what has been driving different societies' need to disempower us. If any of the fears motivating the following examples are true, menstrual blood is the most powerful, badass substance on the planet.

In ancient Egypt, menstrual blood was literally considered sorcery and incorporated into spell casting and medical treatments. In the first century BCE, the Roman naturalist Pliny the Elder claimed that menstrual blood was poisonous, could perform alarming magical feats, and caused wine to sour, trees and crops to die, mirrors to cloud, swords to blunt, and dogs to go mad should they chance to taste it. In primitive societies, menstrual blood was "known" to cure leprosy, warts, birthmarks, gout, hemorrhoids, epilepsy, and headaches.[17] Even as late as 1870, Augustus Kinsley Gardner, the author of *Conjugal Sins Against the Laws of Life and Health*, said that menstrual blood is corrupt and virulent, threatening an unwitting penis with a syndrome now known as gonorrhea.[18] Different eras, same story, eh?

After reading about the magical and mysterious powers of menstrual blood, you can imagine all the reasons menstrual sex has long been deemed a terrible idea. Here are just a few (okay, a ton) of the rules, laws, and prohibitions that further make my point that menstrual blood is some mighty juice.

In the early part of the twentieth century, doctors and psychiatrists perpetuated the myths that women are sexually passive and that they're the least interested in sexual activity while they are menstruating. Kinda weird, since there is plenty of evidence supporting the fact that many women have increased libido during their periods.

Nevertheless, even if your girl wants it, you should probably stay far away when she's on the rag, guys, because nothing but bad is coming your way if you enter that red tent.

Check it out: one South African clan believes that having intercourse with a woman having her period can make a man's bones go soft. In Zoroastrianism, there's a belief that any man who lies with a menstruating woman will beget a demon and be punished in hell by having filth poured into his mouth.[19] The Torah warns against having intercourse with menstruating women because doing so will cause the "cutting of life on earth and the denial of life to come."[20]

Taboos aren't all bad. Historically, they've existed to protect human beings from danger through imagery and storytelling. But this taboo is ironic because, in fact, menstrual intercourse is actually good for the woman—it temporarily relieves cramps by increasing the menstrual flow. And sure, it has long been argued in medical circles that the combination of menstruation and intercourse is harmful to women, but there are absolutely no data to support that.

Given that menstrual blood and having sex with a menstruating woman are so dangerous, you have to wonder, how the hell did we get into this situation where we are so ashamed of such a powerpants showing up once a month? Truthfully, I firmly believe that very early on, we missed a critical opportunity to achieve total world domination. I joke a lot, but I am dead serious here.

It was commonly agreed across eras and cultures that our blood was a source of power, magic, and sorcery. But instead of us using it as our lightsaber, our power tool equipped with unsurpassed power, somehow the whole thing got turned upside down into a super gross, vile, filthy thing to be hidden and ashamed about.

The moment I thought about it like this, a light bulb (yes, another one!) went off and I saw everything about our situation differently. I totally understood why we are where we are and where we need to go in order to make some meaningful changes.

It was what I call a therapeutic revelation. Now, I don't know if you have ever been in therapy or done any group self-improvement work, but sometimes you have a really difficult and/or painful realization. It can happen when you're working with a therapist or doctor and asking "Why am I so sick?" or "Why do I feel so crazy? So depressed? I just don't understand what's going on." Then the others say something like "Well, when you were little, you witnessed something horrible, then your parents had a nasty and violent divorce, or you got mugged in college," and suddenly, even though you knew all of those facts, the impact of the sum of those events comes into focus and you have an *Aha!* moment. You develop a certain amount of newfound compassion for yourself that allows you to begin to transcend your past. You start the process of freeing yourself from the constraints of what has already transpired.

That's how I felt after I learned about the history of the menstrual cycle. It's one of the main motivations behind this book. I want to share how history becomes herstory. I want to finally untangle the shame and association with filth.

So, here's where our story actually begins, through clearly retelling the past, trying to understand its motivations, and deciding that this is the last time that story about women is told— that we seize the opportunity today, right now, to change the way women relate to and experience our periods.

Take Action!

The only way we can change our future is by putting the stories that have constrained and shamed us squarely into the past. Stigma is really a common experience, and a lot of people feel alone in that experience. I'm telling you: you are not alone, and there are things you can do to change the story, for yourself and for other women. Here's an action step that you can do today to start being a change maker.

Tell a woman the history of the menstrual cycle and how it has impacted our present-day relationship with our bodies and the security of our health. Go on Instagram, Twitter, Facebook, and Snapchat, and share the history of how we got here. Or just tell a friend, a sister, your mother, your doctor, your teacher, face-to-face. Sometimes people are shy about doing something publicly, because they don't want to feel even more stigmatized. All of us can act in our own way, depending on our comfort level.

And then tell everyone to stay tuned to learn what we can do about it.

3

·· ·· ·· ··

MANY LIES AND A TRUTH

Reframing the Language and
Stigma Around Periods

In a time of deceit telling the truth is a revolutionary act.

—UNKNOWN

My father used to say it takes two people to tell a lie: one person who doesn't want to know the truth and another who is willing to deliver the lie. Those of us with periods have been pretty much lied to since the beginning of time.

We've been told that periods are a nuisance to be quelled or suppressed, that periods are dirty and filthy, and that the only feelings we should have about them are shame, awkwardness, or embarrassment. The social stigma is such that periods should be tucked away, never to be spoken of because of how truly unclean they are—and, by extension, we are.

The word *period* originates from the Greek roots *peri* and *hodos*, which translate to "around" and "way/path." I think this is incredibly apropos and lovely for something that can reflect our health and guide us toward optimal health. Eventually, that transitioned into the Latin word *periodus,* meaning "recurring cycle." In the 1800s, the English caught on and started calling our cycles "periods," and the rest is history. Since its eloquent origins of meaning "the way" (so very Taoist), attitudes about menstruation have transformed into the polar opposite.

The period tracker Clue, along with the International Women's Health Coalition, did a survey about what people called their periods. This survey received more than 90,000 responses from 190 different countries and reported more than 5,000 euphemisms to describe periods. That study gave us powerful clues about how people (men and women alike) perceived periods. They used words and phrases such as: *on the rag/ragging, red tide/river/sea/moon/light/army/curse/days/dot, code red, bloody Mary, the blob, shark week, red wedding, mad cow disease* (nice), and, of course, *the curse.* It's interesting that there was only one semipositive reference to periods: birthing a blood diamond.[1]

Furthermore, there's an almost universal gag order on the topic of periods or even menstrual blood—we are still seeing pad commercials use that mysterious blue liquid to "represent" blood despite the fact that practically every movie and TV show has so much egregious blood spewing out and no one seems to be upset about that.

Our language or our silence is a direct reflection of our attitudes. We often feel so crazy and sick from our messed-up menstruation that we've forgotten that our monthly bleed is the manifestation of the biological process that can *make a human.*

This little fact has all but been eliminated from the narrative around menstruation, but it's our menstrual blood that makes life for the fertilized embryo possible. Our menstrual blood is critically important in reproduction. Our blood—yes, the scary stuff staining our good panties, the bane of our existence— makes up the maternal placenta that develops from the maternal uterine tissue that makes the uterine lining. And it is our blood that provides the nutrients and oxygen for the developing fetus to grow.

To have shame for what's arguably the most important biological function that ensures the future of our species is, frankly, insane. Loading our periods with allusions to war, attacks, and insanity is dangerous. It creates a taboo around a subject that is vital to the health of women and PWPs that seriously limits our ability to have open, creative conversations about the problems women and PWPs face when dealing with their cycles. The stigma is so universally ingrained in our culture that despite the fact that almost half a billion women every day do not have access to basic menstrual supplies, almost no one knows it—not even other women. When a group of people, namely women and PWPs, experience generational messaging and conditioning that our bodies are shameful and the issues we experience relating to menstruation should be kept hidden away (think menstrual huts), the idea of expressing any needs, concerns, and suffering that have anything to do with our periods becomes unspeakable. When that happens, we end up silently enduring the worst period problems—which we're now convinced are simply what comes with being a woman. (More about why *that* matters later in this chapter.) This stigma runs so deep and so wide that it's nearly invisible.

Most people look at periods as a nuisance, something that just has to be tolerated. We think that if we just ignore our periods, everything will be fine. But let me tell you, periods matter. In fact, I would go so far as to say they matter more than global warming—and that ignoring them puts us into just as much peril. Don't believe me? Think I'm exaggerating? Let me lay out the facts.

We keep ignoring the signs that the planet is deteriorating, and it keeps getting sicker and sicker. We don't believe the changes will affect us in the near term. The impact is already significant, and it will be even more so in the future—for both this generation and future ones. We do the same with our periods. The menstrual cycle is in big trouble, too—the kind that threatens the health and well-being of the majority of women on the planet.

Like the health of our planet, the health of our collective menstrual cycle (and by extension, that means everything from our uteruses to the overall health of all women) is declining. From our menstrual cycles themselves to our fertility to our ability to survive childbirth, the decline is directly caused by human behavior. So, let's take a look at a few indicators of the state of our cycles.

Menstrual Disorders

The number of women diagnosed with menstrual disorders such as endometriosis, PCOS, PMS, and cramping, as well as ovulatory disorders, is staggering.[2]

- Approximately 8 percent of women have PCOS.

- Another 10 percent have endometriosis.

- 84.1 percent (or 55 million) have dysmenorrhea (severe menstrual pain).[3]

- 25.3 percent (16 million) miss school or work even with medication.[4]

- 30 to 40 percent (22.5 million) have significant PMS.[5]

- 13 to 18 percent (10 million) have premenstrual dysphoric disorder (PMDD).[6]

Giving Birth

The safety and quality of giving birth are declining. According to the CDC, in 2017:

- The cesarean delivery rate increased to 32 percent, slightly up from 31.9 percent in 2016; the low-risk cesarean delivery rate increased to 26 percent.

- The rate of preterm births rose for the third year in a row to 9.93 percent.

Despite the fact that the United States spends more on health care than any other country, maternal mortality rates continue to increase—so much so, in fact, that the United Nations has described maternal mortality as a human rights issue at the forefront of US health care. The 2017 NPR and ProPublica series *Lost Mothers: Maternal Mortality in the U.S.* reported that the United States has the highest rate of maternal mortality of any developed country, and it's the only country in which the mortality rate has been rising—to an estimated seven hundred to nine hundred a year.

Our cycles and uteruses are exhibiting the effects of not only our own personal habits but also the slew of chemicals we encounter in everyday living.

- Phthalates (the chemicals added to plastic to make it harden)

- Xenoestrogens (natural chemical compounds that mimic estrogen)

- Bisphenol A (BPA)

- Plastics labeled BPA free

- Dioxin found in nonorganic tampons

- Atrazine found in common weed killer

- Mercury now found in most fish; perfluorinated chemicals

- PFCs found in nonstick cookware and the inside lining of microwave popcorn bags

- Solvents in commercially available cleaning products

These chemicals have a significant impact on our health and the health of our children. Research spanning the last twenty-five years implicates endocrine disruptors like these in many health problems, including male reproductive disorders, premature death, obesity and type 2 diabetes, neurological impacts, breast cancer, endometriosis, female reproductive disorders, immune disorders, liver cancer, osteoporosis, Parkinson's disease symptoms, prostate cancer, thyroid disorders, and more.

When we realize our bodies are constantly bombarded with chemicals that are disabling our reproductive systems, it's incredibly difficult to make headway toward rehabilitating the health and cycles of the individuals (us!) who are exposed to them on a daily basis. So, like our planet, our bodies are suffering and screaming for attention. Both need to have a cleaner environment to be able to thrive.

Common, but Definitely Not at All Normal

Since the beginning of time, women have been told another all-encompassing lie about periods: that PMS cramps, nausea, bloating, emotional roller coasters, breast tenderness, migraines, diarrhea, pain as bad as a heart attack, and all the rest of it are *normal.* They're not symptoms, they're not solvable, they're just the way things are. Our doctors, our friends, even our mothers out-and-out tell us that all this suffering is simply normal.

Think I'm overstating the case? Just to prove it, the team at Brazen partnered with our friends at Thinx period panties and polled 4,000 women about whether they thought PMS and cramping were normal.

A whopping 86 percent thought they were!

But that's simply not true.

We—you!—do not have to feel awful once a month. Let me repeat it: you do not have to—and you *should not*—feel awful every month. Changing the programming around the way we think about our periods is critical to our starting to have agency over our own health. We have continued to believe it's our destiny to suffer—for centuries. It's got to stop. And now is the time for us to transform this conversation from egregious misinformation into an ongoing talk that will help us empower ourselves. A lot of what's going on boils down to the fact that menstrual problems are common—*really* common. But we can't let that confuse this issue. Just because something is common doesn't make it "normal." Common means something that happens frequently or to a lot of people. *Normal* is defined as conforming to a type; a standard, or a regular pattern. And *normal* also means *disease free.* To really get the distinction, let's look at diabetes. Type 2 diabetes is one of the most prevalent diseases today: more than 30 million Americans suffer from it. It is extremely *common,* and getting more so every day, but just because 30 million people have it doesn't mean that it is a *normal* condition for the human body. Rather, it needs to be treated or addressed one way or another—and inaction isn't one of the options.

Menstruation itself is both totally common and totally normal. Menstrual pain is also very common. A full 82 percent of women have significant, life-interrupting PMS and menstrual cramping every month.[7] But it is *not* any more normal than type 2 diabetes and is even more easily correctable. Though the intensity of period pain can vary, significant menstrual pain has been compared to the pain of a heart attack! And remember, pain is a warning sign. It's one way your body tries to tell you that something is wrong or *not* normal—you know, like a heart attack is *not* normal. We ignore pain like that at our peril. Though PMS, cramping, clotting, heavy bleeding, and major mood swings are not necessarily considered a disease in and of themselves, they do indicate that something in your body is not functioning optimally.

Normalizing crappy periods has all kinds of consequences. Women with PMS and PMDD are often misdiagnosed with bipolar disease or other mental illnesses and prescribed antidepressants or lithium, which comes with many unpleasant side effects. Fifteen percent of women with PMDD get so desperate that they attempt to kill themselves—and this is "normal"?

Even so, women have been trained to think all of this menstrual agony *is* normal. You may have been told things such as "Getting cramps is just bad luck," "It's the curse women have to endure because Eve sinned back in the garden of Eden," or even "Cramping is your body training for childbirth." For the record, all of that is complete BS, and it's only the beginning of the ways we've been misled about our periods (for more on that subject, refer back to chapter 2).

Society, authority figures, and even medical professionals are still telling women that unless our problem can be diagnosed as something that Western medicine acknowledges as a "disease"—essentially, something for which there's a medical treatment—it's simply "normal."

It's true that getting sick is a common part of being human. Not doing anything about your pain and sickness? Accepting your suffering as your lot in life? Not even looking for options? None of that is normal—or a good idea. There are no other medical conditions for which we simply accept that pain and suffering are the fate of the patients, no matter how many of them there are or how much they're suffering.

In fact, typically when *80 million people* in the United States have a debilitating condition, no one calls it normal. It's called an *epidemic*.

Your Period Truth

Now to the truth: there is enormous power in what your period is saying to you.

Periods are *the* single most instructive feedback mechanism for your health and fertility. Your menstrual cycle is the canary in your coal mine. Though your blood pressure, cholesterol, and blood sugar level give us important discrete information about various functions of your body, your period is the one tool that arrives on schedule every month to give you a full systems check.

Not only is it incredibly reliable as a diagnostic tool, it costs women—and society—absolutely nothing to use.

What's more, the feedback you get from your period is super detailed. Every aspect of your cycle can give you specific information about how much your body likes or dislikes how you're caring for it. Your period can be:

- Predictive

- Diagnostic

- Prescriptive

What does that mean? It means that if we observe the specific characteristics of our cycles, from the amount of bleeding to the nature and intensity of our PMS symptoms, we can use that information to gauge how easy it will be for us to conceive naturally and stay healthy in the long term. We can learn to read the feedback from our cycles to figure out what physical problems we're facing. And we can use that information to help us create solutions to correct any issues. Learning to understand what your period is telling you is the key to improving how you experience your period, assisting your natural fertility (if that's what you're aiming to do), and potentially reducing the risk of developing major health dangers women face today, such as type 2 diabetes, heart disease, stroke, and estrogen-dependent cancers by significantly improving your overall health.[8, 9]

Every single aspect of your cycle—from how long it lasts and how long you bleed to your specific PMS matrix (Did you know that there are more than fifteen different symptoms associated with PMS? Check out chapter 4 for the full matrix) and the intensity and duration of your PMS, from the color, viscosity, and volume of your menstrual blood to your clotting, cramping, and spotting—can give you an amazingly clear and detailed report card on how your body is functioning.

You may be thinking "Shit! My period is so bad, I must be getting an F in cycle." Don't worry! I'm going to teach you how to interpret all of those signals and create a plan to fix the problems and improve your overall health.

In order to do so, we need to see our periods differently. All of those symptoms, from annoying to downright horrible, are actually incredibly beneficial clues about your health—and what to do about it. What's more, understanding what your period is telling you enables you to do a health check every single month to test the corrections you're making. This will enable you to continue to figure out what your body needs in order to function optimally.

Far from being a curse, this fantastic feedback tool actually gives you a significant unfair advantage over men (at least in terms of access to optimal health) because your cycles enable you to pressure test everything you're doing on a regular basis. For example, say you want to start being a vegan. Go ahead and try it for three months, and watch how your menstrual cycle responds. Do your symptoms improve or get worse? Is your cycle longer or shorter? Are your periods heavier or lighter? Are there any other changes? All that feedback gives you important signals about the impact of your new regimen—and guidance about what to do to continue to fine-tune your health. (We'll get into this in more depth in chapter 6.)

Your period is not your enemy. On the contrary, it's a sound barometer of your overall health.

Reclaiming the Way You Talk and Think About Your Period

So I hope by this point you're starting to come around to the idea that there might be more to our periods than a literal pain in the ass. What's also really important is that ignoring our periods and letting the rest of society ignore them, too, is bad for *all* PWPs— your friends, your sisters, and your daughters. It's bad for every one of the 2.2 billion people on this planet who have periods— and in ways you might not anticipate.

By not talking openly about our cycles, we limit the opportunities for others to understand the impact of our suffering, which prevents us from getting access to solutions to help us. Period stigma is not just about inappropriate remarks or hurt feelings; it has major implications for women's health and how we take care of ourselves. When our society does not treat period stigma as a legitimate form of stigma, it can negatively affect a woman's emotional well-being. For a lot of women, period stigma is a chronic experience, one they experience constantly—from family mem-

bers, doctors, coaches, and partners—whether in the form of period jokes or not getting the menstrual supplies they need, for
example. And it's so easy for women to say, "Oh well, it's my fault
I'm built this way."

Let's see how this plays out.

Self-esteem

When you don't feel well and everyone keeps telling you that
feeling like crap is normal or, worse, that you're hysterical, it can
start to erode your sense of self-worth. I don't know about you,
but most of us already struggle to have positive self-esteem.
Even my most accomplished, fit-as-hell, wise, funny, amazing,
baller friends have a tiny part of themselves that feels as though
they're still somehow not good enough. Perhaps men are more
immune to these inner critics, and research shows that they
have more robust self-esteem than women (though that, too,
is changing), but many women are on an unending mission
to prove that we're good enough. Even though we are already
amazing, somehow many of us can't see or accept it.

Enter the menstrual cycle. Everyone avoids mentioning it,
our blood is feared by all (including ourselves), no one cares that
we feel sick as hell, and the message we get is that society really
prefers that we just go away until the whole thing is over.

That sucks. Because what you think, you become. Where the
mind goes, the body follows.

Let me give you an example of how powerfully your mind
can affect your body. If you had a super cute little kid—I mean the
most awesome, swell child ever—and I came over to your house

and told that kid every day, "You are a stupid little piece of shit," I mean, every day I told that kid a few times how crappy and useless he or she was, how many days or weeks would it take before that child would actually start to become that way? To believe my words so powerfully that his or her mind and body started acting in accordance with my idiotic, made-up, mean story?

Well, the same thing has happened and is happening every day for women! We hear this story perpetuated by the media, by society, by men, and, yes, even by women, all telling us that we're filthy and therefore inferior. And for whatever reason, we believe that shit.

The impact of period silence goes beyond women suffering needlessly. To be healthy and take proper care of themselves, women need clean menstrual supplies such as tampons or pads—but half a *billion* women on the planet don't have access to them. Just take a second to think about that. Half of the population menstruates—and nearly half of *them* don't have the tampons, pads, or even clean clothes they need to take care of their menstrual flow.

This is not a trivial problem. It's impossible to create a society in which all people can have equal access to power when a quarter of them can't get the necessary tools to care for their bodies while they're experiencing a biological function that's absolutely critical for our continued existence as a species.

Education

There's a proverb that says, "If you educate a man, you educate an individual, but if you educate a woman, you educate a nation." I can't overstate how important women's education is. Girls with little or no education are far more likely to be married while they're still children, to suffer domestic violence, to live in poverty, and to lack power over their household spending or even their own health care than are their better-educated peers, according to a new report by the World Bank Group.

In all regions of the world, from Malawi to Manhattan, women who are better educated tend to marry later and have fewer children—and those are good things. "Enhanced agency—the ability to make decisions and act on them—is a key reason why children of better-educated women are less likely to be stunted: "Educated mothers have greater autonomy in making decisions and more power to act for their children's benefit," explains World Bank Group director of gender and development Jeni Klugman in the organization's report. Not only do they earn more money for their families, they take better care of their children and demand a better education for them.

Why am I talking so much about how crucial women's education is? Here's the thing. It's not just about improving our children's lives (though isn't that enough?). In order for women to rise up, we need *access* to education. And there are two very correctable impediments to PWPs going to school. The first one is menstrual pain, which makes it hard for PWPs to focus on school or even attend; the second is absenteeism, which is linked with reduced levels of education.[10]

Access to Power

We all like to think that if people work hard enough, they can overcome anything. This is one of those toxic myths that is perpetuated as the key to success: put in your time, pay your dues, prove yourself. What's worse is that this myth disproportionately affects women. That's BS. In order to have access to power in the education system, workplace, and society, women need education and health care. When women don't have access to menstrual supplies or experience too much pain to go to school or work, they miss out on daily and monthly opportunities to improve their current positions. That's the real glass ceiling, as women don't get the opportunity to lead companies and governments. And thus, the idea that they are inferior, damaged, and/or sick continues to be perpetuated. And it starts early. Only 39 percent of countries have equal proportions of boys and girls enrolled in secondary education.

Knowledge

With that, I'd like to bring this discussion back to *you*. Lack of quality information about our bodies and cycles can damage our future fertility and overall health. Very few women, even those who have been diagnosed, know that issues such as polycystic ovarian syndrome (PCOS) and endometriosis have all been correlated to an increased risk of developing the diseases that are most likely to kill women—such as heart disease, type 2 diabetes, estrogen-dependent cancers, and stroke. Hell, just having significant menstrual cramps associated with endometriosis increases your risk of developing heart disease by 66 percent. You may be thinking "That's too bizarre! How are my cramps related to my heart?" I'm so glad you asked that question! It's the beginning of your entrée into the world of *everything is connected*.

If you have bad menstrual cramps, you probably know that they're often associated with menstrual clotting—you know, the thick clumps of blood you find on your tampon or pad, or in your cup. Well, if the blood tends to coagulate in your uterus, conditions that are causing that are likely also impacting blood flow in your other organs, such as your heart, and making clots more likely there as well. This is just one example of how the systems of your body are connected—and why your period can tell you so much about the rest of your body—but it's a theme I'll return to often and explain further. In the next chapter, we'll dive into the signs and signals your period is trying to communicate to you— and what exactly they can tell you.

CASE STUDY

CHANGING THE CONVERSATION

We can't understand what our periods mean to us and our overall health until we can think about them without all the misconceptions that blind us. Let the following story serve as an example.

Recently I spoke with a woman who has a 17-year-old daughter. The mom said to me in the most apologetic tone, "I don't want to sound like I'm whining, but my daughter is really in trouble. She has been so depressed and even cuts herself when she gets really low." (As if her concern could be called "whining"!) "She has been on a ton of meds, which seem to make her worse. We've been to so many doctors. But here's the thing. I think it's tied to her menstrual cycle. This probably sounds crazy, but she seems exponentially better—until she ovulates, and then the shit hits the fan."

She went on to tell me that her daughter's doctors didn't think that her depression was related to her cycle. The final straw: the doctors had tried yet another medication, and that time the young woman had had a nearly fatal reaction to the drug and had ended up in the ER. At the end of her rope, the mother had come to me.

Immediately, I thought that this young woman didn't actually have bipolar disorder but rather probably had premenstrual dysphoric disorder (PMDD), the very severe form of PMS. I asked her if the doctors had looked into that, and she said she had never heard of PMDD even though they had been going to various doctors for three years about her daughter's condition. I suggested we do a test to see if her emotional symptoms would respond to my Chinese herbal formula for PMS, which improves the ability of the liver to break down and metabolize hormones. I told her that if it helped at all, it could be an indicator that her daughter had more of a hormonal problem than a chemical/psychological issue.

Often Chinese medicine sees organ function differently from Western medicine, and if you have experience understanding your body only from that point of view, the Chinese medicine approach can seem foreign—and hard to buy into. In Western medicine, one of the jobs of the liver is to metabolize or break down hormones. Chinese and Western medicine agree on this. But the Chinese take it a step further. They also think the liver is responsible for the smooth movement of *everything*. When I say "everything," I mean hormone balance, blood (including circulation), energy, and even emotions. When the liver is working optimally, all of those systems will be working well. There won't be PMS/PMDD, there won't be clotting or cramping, emotions will be balanced. But when the liver isn't functioning, Chinese medicine says it is stagnant, and one of the most common symptoms associated with liver stagnation is depression.

Two weeks later, the mother called me back crying. I was so worried that something terrible had happened, as I knew she was concerned about the daughter's safety. When I asked her what had happened, she exclaimed, "She didn't cut herself once this month!" I asked her how much better she was, and she said, "At least seventy percent, which is *huge* for us. She is still acting like a seventeen-year-old bitchy teenager, but we are so happy for that! That's normal."

This is a perfect example of how both our attitudes about our cycles and our lack of understanding of what they're telling us contribute to our suffering.

Take Action!

Go to https://foreverbrazen.com/pages/manifesto and join the Menstrual Defense Fund, where you can learn how to get involved.

4

....

HOW TO READ YOUR PERIOD

One of the most sincere forms of respect is actually
listening to what another has to say.

—BRYANT H. MCGILL

All day, every day, your body is communicating with you. There are many messages that we eagerly respond to, such as hunger pangs (cake, anyone?). Or the drowsiness inviting us to sleep, or even the urge to have a BM. These are signals we almost never ignore, but beyond these signals, our bodies are communicating with cells, tissues, organs, nervous systems, endocrine systems, and our brain. More important, your period is communicating with you every day of your cycle, giving you robust and valuable feedback. We have basically been trained to ignore these signals, and now, for many women, our cycles are screaming at us, demanding to be heard. Our bodies are in desperate need of support and respect, but they're calling for help in a way that few of us can comprehend. In this chapter, I'm going to deconstruct some of this mysterious language to help you understand what your period is telling you.

For the last twenty years, I've been working with women who were struggling to get pregnant. People always ask me what the best strategies are to improve fertility outcomes. Most commonly they ask, "What are the herbs and foods that are best for fertility?"

I always answer, "Nothing. No matter what you read, there are no foods or herbs that are going to make you fertile!"

The absolute best thing that you can do to improve your fertility—or period or *health*—is to figure out all of what's wrong and attend to *everything*. Whatever's happening with your uterus or ovaries is just a symptom of a bunch of other problems. Infertility is a by-product of diet, lifestyle, environment, habits, and exposure to stress, as well as how your body responds to them. If you can understand what's wrong with your menstrual cycle, your habits, and the signs and symptoms that are contributing to your inability to get pregnant, then you'll start to get some real answers. The secret is in the intersection of all of these factors.

The Ideal Cycle

Over the years, thousands of women have sought out my help to improve their fertility and menstrual cycles. When I began the work, almost as soon as their first visit, I noticed that their menstrual cycles were substandard in virtually every way. Short cycles, long cycles, PMS, cramping, heavy bleeding, irregular ovulation and cycle patterns—and the graphs of their basal body temperature looked like random squiggles instead of smooth reflections of hormonal balance. I also noticed that most of them were under tremendous pressure and stress in their lives, meaning that a lot of their habits weren't likely to keep their bodies healthy.

As I worked with those women, using the menstrual cycle as a quantifiable diagnostic tool and as a driver of the kinds of treatments I delivered, each patient's entire menstrual cycle, basal body temperatures, and habits started to improve. Typically, the menstrual cycle got better over a period of about three months. The patient's PMS and cramps became almost nonexistent. If she had too much bleeding, the period length reduced to closer to four days; or if she didn't have enough blood and therefore had a short period, the period duration increased to closer to four days. The color of her menstrual blood looked fresher and redder instead of pink or dark. Her ovulation started to become more regular. She had healthier cervical discharge, and her temperature graphs started smoothing out. All of those functions improved until the woman reached a state in which she could get pregnant naturally, even if she'd previously been infertile.

At some point, probably around seven years into my clinical practice, I realized that the menstrual pattern that they were achieving is the ideal formula for fertility and for health. When their cycles reached that point, they had a very high incidence of natural pregnancy and significant improvements in IVF outcomes. It became such a reliable barometer of natural fertility that I started to aspire to it for my patients.

This ideal menstrual cycle may seem like a unicorn—it sounds beautiful, but hardly anyone has seen it, if it exists at all—but the reality is, at least in my clinical practice, that about 80 percent of women, no matter their starting point, were able to get fairly close to the ideal state. It doesn't happen by magic, but a "perfect" cycle is possible if you work to identify what the issues are and create a precise intervention that uses diet, lifestyle, mindfulness and mind-set training, stress management, and prescriptive Chinese herbs.

Let me tell you what an ideal menstrual cycle looks like. Remember, this is *not* a unicorn. This is a totally achievable cycle for most women.

The ideal menstrual cycle is twenty-eight days long, with ovulation on the fourteenth day of the cycle with healthy cervical discharge that's stretchy and clear. Throughout the cycle, there's no PMS, no cramping, no clotting, and no spotting between periods, and when the menstrual blood comes, it's fresh and red. There's enough blood to soak a tampon or a pad every four hours for four days, neither more nor less.

There you have it. Easy, right? In this chapter, I'm going to tell you all about each of the elements that I described.

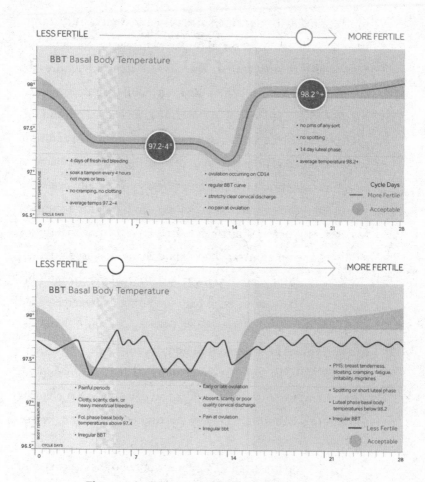

These graphs illustrate the different phases of your cycle.
(Illustrations courtesy of the author)

Before we get into the nitty-gritty, I think it's important to explain a little more about how most of us have been trained to look at our bodies through the lens of Western medicine. Basically, we've been taught to think each individual symptom or problem we experience occurs in isolation and therefore we should treat it in isolation. Though this is a very straightforward approach to medicine, since so many women are sick from their periods, we know that it isn't working very well for us—or anyone else, for that matter. This myopic approach ignores the fact that every organ system and our habits are deeply interconnected. We fail to look at the body as an ecosystem and forget to recognize how this system affects our health. In addition, we tend to neglect the idea of implementing systemic changes, which can significantly affect our health. Typically, we see a symptom—such as achy knee joints—and look for a solution to correct it, such as a pill or an exercise. We assume that there's a one-to-one relationship. A systemic change is based on identifying a symptom and tracking it back to what may be multiple sources, in the case of knee pain including overexercise, bad walking form, low collagen level, overweight—and that's just the beginning. In order to best address any issue, you have to identify all the factors that contribute to it and start to work on all of them in steps. Then you can achieve quantum changes in both the symptom you were starting with and your whole system.

I'd like you to start thinking about your body as an ecosystem in which everything—from all the organs to what you eat, from how much you sleep to how you manage stress, from your temperatures to your aches and pains—feeds into the dynamic. I want to emphasize the importance of how the elements within your ecosystem interact, producing the side effect that is your health. As you read this book, you'll see the many ways this concept plays out and how viewing things this way can help you take more control of your health and well-being.

• • •

Okay, *now* let's talk about each individual part of your menstrual cycle that you can use to better understand your overall health.

We'll be looking at:

- The functions of blood

- The color of your menstrual blood

- The volume of your menstrual blood

- The quality of your menstrual blood

- The length of your cycle

- Your cervical discharge

- Your PMS

The Functions of Blood

In general, your blood is vital for almost every function in your body, and it has several different jobs:

1. It supplies oxygen and nutrients, including amino acids and glucose, to every cell in your body, including those in the brain, muscles, organs, and tissues.

2. It transports not just nutrients but also hormones and messages throughout your body. Without blood, hormonal cycles such as ovulation would not occur.

3. It regulates body temperature. On the one hand, it can have a cooling function by moving warmth away from your internal organs to the capillaries near the surface of your skin. On the other, it can carry warmth to extremities that have been overcooled by the environment.

4. It removes and transports wastes including carbon dioxide, urea, and lactic acid so you can properly eliminate them. For example, it moves carbon dioxide from the tissues and organs into the lungs to be exhaled.

5. It supports immune function, and it takes protective action against disease. White blood cells defend the body against infections, foreign materials, and abnormal cells.

6. It works to regulate body acidity (pH level).

7. It engorges parts of the body when needed, causing, for example, a penile erection or your clitoris's response to sexual arousal (which, incidentally, is omitted from almost every source that discusses this function of blood).

8. It transports clotting agents to the site of a hemorrhage. The platelets in blood enable clotting, or coagulation.

When bleeding occurs, platelets group together to create a clot. The clot then becomes a scab and stops the bleeding.

But what exactly is menstrual blood?

Menstrual blood is made up of thickened endometrial cells that slough off monthly if you're not pregnant, together with arterial blood from the arteries that feed the uterus and some clots. Most doctors will tell you that clotting is normal and in fact demonstrates that your body has the ability to slow down your bleeding if it is too heavy. Part of this is true. You do want your body to be able to shore up unchecked bleeding, but I disagree with the idea that it's *normal*. This falls into the category of "common but not normal." The concept fails to consider the question "Why is there unchecked bleeding, and is that normal?" No, of course not. When you identify the problem that is causing the heavy bleeding and improve healthy blood flow (I use Chinese herbs to do this), the clots and heavy flow go away, and you know what else? So does cramping.

CHINESE HERBS

How do herbs work to improve cramping, clotting, and heavy bleeding? First, it is important to know that an acupuncturist almost never uses just one herb. No one herb can fix everything. The trick to using herbs is central to everything you are reading in this book: to stop cramping and heavy bleeding, you have to look at all the systems that work together, including the following.

1. Blood needs to circulate freely. When this is happening, your menstrual blood will be a fresh red color with no clotting (and hence no cramping).

2. Your temperature needs to be neither too hot nor too cold. Cold causes the blood to stagnate (think what happens when water freezes), and heat causes too much bleeding (think Ebola—but not as bad, obviously).

3. Your liver has to be able to metabolize hormones and regulate blood flow.

So how can we address this? We build formulas with very precise doses and ingredients to address all of these causes. When there is precision in both the ingredients and doses tailored to the patient's specific root cause, we don't have to worry about addressing each individual symptom.

Your menstrual blood is one reflection of your uterine lining and overall health. Its quality is an important factor in IVF outcomes,[1] fetal birth-weight outcomes,[2] and the risk of ectopic pregnancies.[3] If you think about all of your symptoms as measures of how well your body is performing overall, the volume and quality of your menstrual blood is a measure of the quality of the food you're eating and your body's ability to break it down, extract the nutrients, and turn them into energy to make bone marrow, which then makes blood, which then supports building a healthy uterine lining and finally expelling it as your menstrual blood.

The Color of Your Menstrual Blood

You might think the color of your menstrual blood is insignificant, but according to the principles of traditional Chinese medicine, we can learn a lot from it. As I said before, we are trained to think that each physical symptom is encapsulated in one part of the body, but your menstrual blood gives you a peek at how your body is managing your blood *everywhere*. It's a wonderful barometer of the density of your red blood cells, your level of blood oxidation, and how well your blood is flowing. Let's look at the different colors.

- **Fresh red.** This is what you want. Fresh red is the ideal color for blood. When your menstrual blood is bright red, it means that you're capable of taking the food you're eating and successfully converting it into high-quality blood that fulfills its function in your body. It has a high level of iron and is moving freely through your circulatory system. This is critical to good overall health because blood carries oxygen and nutrients to every cell, tissue, and organ in your body. When the quantity and/ or quality is low, every system will suffer.

- **Pink.** Light-colored menstrual blood looks pink because it has fewer red blood cells in it than fresh red blood does. It's really important to pay attention to pink blood because it indicates a deficiency in the concentration of red blood cells. This is different from Western medicine's clinical diagnosis of anemia. Anemia is a deficiency of red blood cells overall, while the Chinese medicine version is more like a low mean corpuscular volume (MCV). When PWPs have light-colored blood, there are often other symptoms as well, such as anxiety, insomnia, and PMS. The deficiency of red blood cells may be caused by a digestive issue in which your body is struggling to extract nutrients from the food you eat, or the quality and/or quantity of your diet may be insufficient to produce abundant, high-quality blood.

- **Rusty.** When menstrual blood appears more brown than red, it indicates that the blood is old and stagnant. It isn't moving freely through your blood vessels, and because of this, it appears oxidized. Often women with rusty blood have early ovulation and higher-than-average temperatures in the follicular phase (cycle days 1 to 14, the first two weeks after bleeding starts).

- **Purple.** Dark or purple blood indicates that the blood is thicker than you want it to be and *really* stagnant— meaning it is more viscous than what you would see when you cut yourself. This kind of blood is associated with the feeling of pain and cramping during your period. This is also associated with an increased risk of cardiovascular disease. Recent studies have shown blood viscosity was elevated in patients who experienced cardiovascular events (ischemic heart attacks and strokes) relative to those who did not. Why? Though the quality of your menstrual blood isn't a direct analogue to your circulating blood, it is an excellent close correlate. You can assume that if your menstrual blood is dark and clotted, your circulating blood is also more coagulated and viscous, which isn't good for your body and especially not for your heart.

- **Black.** This is bad. This is basically purple blood on crack, and you are certainly going to experience significant pain during your period. In my experience, women with very dark purple or black blood have a very high incidence of fibroids. I have seen this improve only with potent herb combinations like the ones in our Brazen supplement formula, which dissolve the old, stuck blood and improve circulation. A combination of fennel seed, ginger root, curcumin, and motherwort relaxes spasms, improves circulation, and decreases pain.

The Volume of Your Menstrual Blood

In the same way that the color of your blood gives you information about your overall health, the volume of your blood can also be used diagnostically. Studies show that menstrual bleeding volume is correlated with IVF success, for instance. You may be thinking "But I don't want to get pregnant, I just want to fix my period and get healthy." That's totally fine, but when we think about your fertility as an expression of your optimal health, we can look at the factors that have been shown to significantly impact fertility to validate the optimal state of overall health you're working toward. In a small pilot study at Conceivable of 105 women, we found that the closer women got to having the ideal menstrual cycle, the more likely they were to get pregnant—even if they had been previously diagnosed as infertile. There wasn't one factor that had more weight in its ability to increase natural fertility outcomes, rather, it was the combination of the whole system that appeared to make the biggest difference. We have found that women experiencing fewer than four days of bleeding soaking a tampon or pad or filling a cup every four hours are less likely to have successful IVF cycles and more likely to have challenges producing a uterine lining sufficient for implantation. Sometimes you may have more than four days of bleeding and/or soak more than a tampon or pad or fill a cup every four hours. We often think that more is better, but this concept gets us into lots of trouble. We think that exercising more is better, being skinnier is better, drinking more wine is *always* better (just kidding), working longer hours is better—so, of course, it would be better to have more than the ideal amount of blood, right? Not so much. Look, sisters, I can assure you of this as a recovering type A overachieving person who wore myself out so intensively that my legs stopped working, I also thought that more was better, but it almost never is. The right amount is the right amount. Too much is pathological (meaning that there is a problem), and too little is also pathological. More than four days every four hours is almost always accompanied by clotting, which may be restraining the bleeding necessary to release your old uterine lining. Insufficient blood flow indicates either that your digestion can't break food down efficiently and turn it into bone marrow and then blood or that the quality and/or quantity of your diet isn't enough to make high-quality blood.

The Quality of Your Menstrual Blood aka Clotting

The job of clots is to slow down your menstrual bleeding so you don't bleed out if the flow is too great. That seems like a really good and important function, right? But let me ask you, have you ever noticed that when you have clotting, it's typically associated with pain and heavy bleeding, but when the bleeding slows down, your pain becomes almost nonexistent?

Conventionally, we think that heavy bleeding causes clotting, but in my opinion (based on my clinical experience), the opposite is true: clotting is the body's mechanism to stop bleeding.

See, your period starts when hormones trigger your body to shed your uterine lining. When this happens, the small blood vessels are exposed, and they bleed. As the blood pools in your uterus, it triggers the release of anticoagulants to help break down the blood and tissues so you can pass them out of your cervix, but when you are having really heavy bleeding, your body may not be able to produce adequate amounts of anticoagulants and you will start seeing clots. You will also read online that this is perfectly normal unless you have really large clots or hemorrhagic (really heavy) bleeding, but again, though this is very common, it is not normal.

By assuming this is normal, we miss a subtle clue that although something isn't actually wrong, it isn't really right, either. Why else do some women have no clots and moderate bleeding? Luck? Seriously, I have heard that exact lame guess as the most common response. But if you look carefully, you will see very common patterns associated with clotting in menstrual blood that are excellent cues for which areas in your body need support.

According to traditional Chinese medicine, the main three things that contribute to clotting (and cramping) are low body temperature, weak digestive function (transformation of food into energy) issues, and blood deficiency. You will also notice that once you get rid of the clots, you will often shed almost no blood in your next cycle or two. Frequently women go from five to six days of heavy bleeding, clotting, and cramping to only one to two days of bleeding. In other words, they typically go from having very heavy bleeding to having very scanty bleeding before their periods become regular. That's because their resources have become so depleted that their bodies need to recover and regroup before they can produce a more ideal period.

The Length of Your Cycle

Data show that an ideal cycle for optimal fertility is twenty-eight to thirty days. Here's why: most women think that variability in how long they go between periods is normal. But as we've said before, just because most women have variable cycles doesn't mean that they're normal or, more important, healthy, which is what we're shooting for.

When your period-to-period cycle is between twenty-eight and thirty days, the follicle (unfertilized egg) has the perfect amount of time to mature. When your cycle is less than twenty-six days, your likelihood of conception is decreased by 50 percent (and, as we've discussed already, your fertility can be an important indicator of your general health). This is because ovulation occurs earlier and the follicle is more immature than is ideal. This is really important because your body is designed to ripen the egg so that it's perfectly primed for fertilization at cycle day 14.

When your cycle is more than thirty-two days long, the follicle is not released until cycle day 16 or later, which makes it less viable for fertilization. A longer cycle is often associated with irregular ovulation and PCOS. Often there is a high correlation between an irregular cycle and PMS,[4] as well. One of the functions of your liver is to metabolize or break down hormones and help your body remove them. When the liver isn't functioning well enough, its ability to regulate the hormones necessary to produce a regular cycle is also disrupted. This can cause hormonal side effects like acne, mood swings, and bloating.

Your Cervical Discharge

That clear, stretchy goop you find in your panties once in a while has a name—cervical mucus—and a lot of important functions. For starters, it keeps your vagina lubricated and healthy. What is also important if you're trying to get pregnant is that it provides the ladder through which sperm swim to get from your vagina into your uterus.

Cervical mucus is also important for the following reasons:

1. It protects the sperm from the hostile vaginal environment. Remember, the vagina is filled with bacteria that are designed to keep the reproductive system safe from intruders. Without good-quality cervical mucus, the sperm cannot survive.

2. It's like a security system to screen and eliminate genetically malformed or abnormal sperm, and it ensures that the remaining sperm's surfaces are clean.

3. It provides biochemical support for the sperm in preparation for fertilization of the egg. See, we are still taking care of the men.

4. It can also store the sperm for later release to coordinate with the best time for insemination with the egg. Your window of fertility is six days, and the sperm can live (with the help of the cervical mucus) for four days.

Like the other features of your cycle, your cervical mucus can vary a lot, and each variation signals different things about your health.

- **Clear and stretchy.** This is the one you want, ideally. It signals that everything is in working order.

- **White.** A thick white discharge when you're *not* ovulating is normal. But if you have any itching or burning, you could have a yeast infection.

- **Yellow or green.** This type of discharge is never normal. It usually indicates a yeast or bacterial infection or possibly a sexually transmitted disease.

- **Brown.** This color is also abnormal. It's often associated with irregular cycles caused by leftover blood in the uterus. However, if you have this frequently, it's best to talk to your doctor, as it can sometimes be a sign of cancer.

- **None.** This isn't usually on discharge lists, but it's an important one to watch if you're trying to get pregnant or even thinking about getting pregnant in the future. Your discharge, like your period, is a reflection of how your body and cycle are working. Sperm need cervical mucus to travel from your vagina to your uterus. You might be thinking "Well, I can use an artificial mucus that seems to work fine." That kind of product does work well to help the transit of sperm, but you'd be missing the chance to figure out and fix a symptom that's telling you that something is out of whack in your body's ecosystem.

Your PMS

Your PMS can tell you a whole lot about yourself—and no, not just that you're feeling so bitchy! The specific symptoms you typically get can reveal all kinds of information about your health.

Let's start with the basics.

What is PMS? It's a combination of physical and emotional symptoms. Research has shown that more than 90 percent of PWPs get some premenstrual symptoms, which can include bloating, headaches, and moodiness. And 5 percent of women of childbearing age have the more severe form of PMS, PMDD. According to the Mayo Clinic, PMDD is a severe, sometimes disabling extension of PMS and often causes extreme mood shifts that can disrupt your work and damage your relationships.

PMS can last from several days to two weeks and typically goes away a few days after your period starts and your hormone levels begin rising again. Often people (both men and women) think that PMS is something to be tolerated rather than a health issue, but it can be quite significant and impactful for the large numbers of women who experience it. Many women have such severe PMS that even everyday activities such as going to work or school can become incredibly difficult. It can also be a real strain on relationships. I spoke with a couple recently who were both extremely concerned with the impact her PMS was having on their quality of life together. He said he felt stressed because he was so nervous worrying about setting her off. He felt as though he had to walk on eggshells for half of the month and then she would come back to him again after she had her period. She was crying the whole time we were talking. She said she knew she was being horrible to him, but she just couldn't change her mood or behavior until after her period. Life-interrupting PMS symptoms such as these may be a sign of PMDD, which can be so debilitating that approximately 15 percent of women with PMDD attempt suicide at least once in their lives.

PMS is seen more frequently in women with high levels of stress and a family history of depression—or a personal history of either postpartum depression or depression.[5]

PMS often starts when women are just beginning their reproductive journey, and unfortunately they are told to just try to grind it out, missing the opportunity to use the signs and symptoms as signals that something is actually wrong. Their symptoms can be quite severe but occasionally improve until they go into perimenopause, when it can start all over again. Joy.

What causes PMS? Through the lens of Western medicine, the cause of PMS is unclear, although some researchers hypothesize that it's related to sensitivity to our fluctuating hormones, which may be associated with how well the liver is metabolizing and excreting hormones.

PMS symptoms can be divided into two basic groups, physical and emotional. Physical symptoms of PMS include:[6]

- Cramping

- Appetite changes or food cravings

- Swollen or tender breasts

- Constipation or diarrhea

- Bloating or a gassy feeling

- Headache or backache

- Clumsiness

- Lower tolerance for noise or light

- Migraine

Emotional or mental symptoms of PMS include:

- Irritability or hostile behavior

- Tension or anxiety

- Depression, feelings of sadness, or crying spells

- Mood swings

- Less interest in sex

- Feeling tired

- Sleep problems (sleeping too much or too little)

- Trouble with concentration or memory

It's important to understand how dramatically your ability or inability to metabolize your hormones can affect your whole system. More than 50 percent of women who experience significant PMS also have another health problem that often gets worse between ovulation and their period.[7] (I hope you're starting to see why I'm so obsessed with how everything is connected!) These conditions often share many symptoms with PMS. They include:

- **Depression and anxiety disorders.** These are the most common conditions that overlap with PMS. The symptoms of depression and anxiety are similar to many PMS symptoms and may get worse before or during your period.

- **Myalgic encephalomyelitis/chronic fatigue syndrome (ME/CFS).** Some women report that their ME/CFS symptoms get worse right before their periods. And research shows that women with ME/CFS may also be more likely to have heavy menstrual bleeding and early or premature menopause.

- **Irritable bowel syndrome (IBS).** IBS causes cramping, bloating, and gas. If you have IBS, your symptoms may get worse right before your period.

- **Bladder pain syndrome.** Women with bladder pain syndrome are more likely to have painful cramps during PMS.

PMS may also worsen some health problems, such as asthma, allergies, and migraines.

I often see articles that ask how PMS can be diagnosed. It's pretty clear to me: if you have any of the aforementioned symptoms between ovulation and your period and the symptoms go away as soon as you start bleeding—it's probably PMS. If you have any concerns about it, be sure to discuss your symptoms with your doctor.

The Importance of Tracking

There are hundreds of period trackers that help you track your temperature, both online and off. If you're trying to get pregnant, you're probably using one of them, such as Clue or Glow, already. Many, many women track their periods, even if they're not trying to get pregnant. That always seemed astonishing to me, but whenever I've asked women why they track, they tell me that they want to know more about their periods. They want to know when they're going to menstruate and even when they're ovulating—either to help prevent unwanted pregnancy or to time sex with their ovulation so that they can increase their chances of getting pregnant. Even beyond those practicalities, these women have a sense that their periods are an integral part of their health, but they don't know exactly how all the pieces fit together.

Tracking is great to help you increase your awareness of how your body is working and give you data. But it can do only so much for you. If you're one of the PWPs who track, there are some important facts to know about what a traditional tracker can and can't do.

A traditional tracker is excellent at collecting your data to predict when you'll be ovulating and when you'll be menstruating. It's easy to use a tracker for this, and the data can be invaluable for you if you're trying to get pregnant. But a tracker can't change or improve your period. It can't explain the deep relationship between your habits and your symptoms and how they're all being reflected in your menstrual cycle. And it can't use your temperatures diagnostically to improve your health.

Tracking and understanding cycle elements like cycle length, color and volume of your blood, pain, and presence of clotting will help you start to see beyond the individual symptoms. Once you can see your cycle as representative of your whole personal ecosystem, you can start to push various levers toward more global outcomes. Instead of just improving a symptom that is impacting your life every month, you can use the various signs and symptoms as guideposts to changing every aspect of your health and start to kick ass like never before.

What kinds of things should you be tracking?

In my opinion, people are tracking way too many things. You want to track things that can actually inform your future behavior. Otherwise, it's more useless data that often stress you out because you don't know how to change them.

What should you track? You should track the number of days

in your cycle, the number of days of bleeding, how long it takes to soak what you use, the kind and intensity of your PMS, the number of days of cramping, and the intensity of menstrual pain. These are the main symptoms that will improve with behavioral and dietary changes in order to give you a sense of how your body is working.

If you're trying to get pregnant, add cervical discharge and basal temperatures because they can be very valuable diagnostically.

TAKE ACTION!

Whether it is on an app or just on the back on a napkin, start tracking your cycle. Knowledge is power.

5
· · · · · · · · · ·

HOW TO BIOHACK
YOUR PERIOD, PART 1

Medicine and Technology

*You are the sum total of everything you've ever seen,
heard, eaten, smelled, been told, forgot—it's all there.
Everything influences each of us, and because of that, I
try to make sure that my experiences are positive.*

—MAYA ANGELOU

When it comes to your menstrual cycle, what does *biohack* mean?

I am not sure I ever met a woman who loved her period. Most of us just want it to go away and stop ruining our best underpants. We don't really think about "fixing" our periods, mostly because we aren't aware that there *is* a fix. We are pretty convinced that this is our screwed-up lot in life and we'd better arm ourselves with the best of what is available to weather the storm and hope that we don't drive our partners away. But the fix isn't taking acetaminophen or taking birth control, although both can help in some cases. It is really about two things: first, changing the conversation about our periods and embracing period power, and second, changing our habits and environment so we can better manage our own biology. Women are excellent biohackers! You're already doing it if you're tracking your cycle for the best time to get pregnant or using birth control to manage your hormones.

Most women don't want to just survive their periods, but they just don't think there is anything that can really make a difference. Many use acetaminophen—even though, according to the black-box warning on the package, you should not exceed 4,000 milligrams within a twenty-four-hour period, or take with more than three alcoholic drinks a day to manage it without risking significant side effects such as liver damage.[1] To curb PMS, we also use Midol, which is just acetaminophen plus caffeine and a diuretic to reduce bloating. We use hot-water bottles and heating pads. We use pot tampons and suppositories—I still haven't figured out how to keep the goo in my vagina when I go to work! We even use TENS units (TENS stands for transcutaneous electrical nerve stimulation—scary, right?) to gently shock our uteri into submission. We are very good at coming up with ways to bandage our pain so we can survive another month.

Let's look at what we are currently using to survive our cycles.

Oral Contraception aka "The Pill"

At this point you may be saying "Bring on the Band-Aids! Fixing my period seems like a pain in the butt to try to figure out. I can just take birth control pills, and that will make most of my symptoms better. Basically, I'll just take a little blue pill, and, like magic, my problems will evaporate. Why not?" Almost one in three women take the pill because they've been advised that it will regulate their periods, according to the 2018 National Survey of Family Growth (NSFG). Menstrual-related disorders and irregular periods are particularly common during adolescence, so it's not surprising that the study found that teens aged 15 to 19 who use the pill are more likely to do so at least partly for noncontraceptive purposes (82%) than for birth control (67%). Moreover, 33 percent of all teens who take the pill report using oral contraceptives solely for noncontraceptive purposes.[2]

And it's not just teens. The survey also revealed that after pregnancy prevention (86%), the most common reasons women of all ages use the pill include reducing cramps or menstrual pain (31%); menstrual regulation, which for some women may help prevent migraines and other painful "side effects" of menstruation (28%); treatment of acne (14%); and treatment of endometriosis (4%). Additionally, it found that some 762,000 women who have never had sex use the pill, and they do so almost exclusively (99%) for noncontraceptive reasons.[3]

So, women are using the pill to suppress their periods in the hope of controlling symptoms such as PMS, cramps, anxiety, heavy bleeding, and irregular cycles and it can be very effective at controlling symptoms if that is what you are after. Although oral contraception will improve some of these symptoms, it's masking symptoms that may be indicators that something more serious is going on, and, more important, the underlying causes of those symptoms that may actually be correctable.

Don't get me wrong, I love oral contraception. Especially when it's used for, well, contraception, which it makes easy and effective. There are absolutely other legit uses for it, too. In a study in conjunction with the Guttmacher Institute exploring the incidence and impact of prescribing oral contraceptives for menstrual management, Rachel K. Jones showed that there are a number of other important health reasons why oral contraceptives should be readily available to the millions of women who rely on them each year.[4] That and other studies have shown how contraceptives can "control" some of the more bothersome symptoms, such as:[5]

- Dysmenorrhea

- Menstrual migraine

- PMS

- Menorrhagia (super-heavy periods)

- Ovarian cysts

- Endometriosis

- Pelvic pain

What the reports don't say is that these conditions have also been shown to respond to modifiable lifestyle factors such as diet, exercise, stress management, and herbal supplementation. Using oral contraceptives to "fix" your period may be the fastest, most readily available solution, but it may not be in your best interest. Women often assume that oral contraceptives have a corrective effect on their period problems since their symptoms get much better when their cycles are suppressed. But this is not the case, as you can see from the data below that Holly Grigg-Spall, the author of *Sweetening the Pill: Or How We Got Hooked on Hormonal Birth Control*,[6] shared in her recent article "Nine Major Myths about the Pill—From Cancer to Weight Gain":[7]

- **Depression.** Taking oral contraception can increase your chances of depression and even suicide. Two large-scale studies from the University of Copenhagen have revealed that for users of the combined pill, the likelihood of a diagnosis of depression is increased by 23 percent, and for users of all hormonal contraceptive types, the risk of suicide is increased threefold. And for teenage women, the diagnosis of clinical depression is 80 percent higher and the suicide risk doubles after just one year of use.

- **Cancer.** For women who use the pill for a decade or longer, a systematic review of twenty-eight scientific studies revealed that the risk of cervical cancer doubles; and a study of 1.8 million women showed that the risk of breast cancer increases by 38 percent.

- **Blood clots.** Many newer contraceptives carry a higher risk of developing blood clots—and their potentially serious or even fatal complications—than do older combined oral contraceptives. Let me be clear: you are at elevated risk on any pill if you are overweight, over thirty-five, or a smoker—but you are also at far higher risk if you have factor V Leiden, an inherited blood-clotting disorder that is considered very common. The risk is high enough that, personally, if I were going to start taking birth control (and especially if I had any other risk factors), I would request that my doctor check to make sure I did not have factor V Leiden before I started taking them so that I could fully understand my risk. This is a simple blood test that you can request from your doctor.

- **Fertility.** Some women are under the misconception that taking hormonal birth control actually preserves your fertility by preventing ovulation. It's a logical conclusion since we're born with all of our eggs and preventing ovulation could be a means of extending our fertile lives. But the data simply do not support this, and being on the pill can affect your fertility in multiple ways, including:

  - **AMH.** In addition to menstrual issues getting worse while suppressed by oral contraceptives, research shows that they can impact the level of anti-Müllerian hormone (AMH), a hormone that's

measured to assess fertility. It gives an approxima-
tion of the number of follicles (unfertilized eggs)
you have. If that number goes down as a result of
taking oral contraceptives, you could infer that the
pill may be reducing your overall fertility.

- **Uterine health.** Additionally, long-term oral contraceptives have been linked with a thin uterine lining, something that can significantly impact your
  ability to both become and stay pregnant.

- **Absorption of essential vitamins and minerals.**
  Last, taking the pill can significantly impact your
  absorption of vitamins and minerals that are essential for regular ovulation, as well as conceiving
  and sustaining a pregnancy, which is probably why
  there is the abovementioned concurrent side effect
  of decreased uterine lining. Remember, if you can't
  break down the food you are eating, turn it into energy, and absorb it to make the building blocks of
  bone marrow, you aren't going to be making much
  of a uterine lining, either.

The bottom line is this: we think of oral contraceptives as
a temporary fix for both our menstrual issues and our desire to
prevent unwanted pregnancy, but unfortunately both come with
risks and side effects most women are unaware of.

Pain Relievers

There are over-the-counter and prescription medicines that can help treat some PMS and menstrual pain symptoms. Pain relievers you can buy in most drugstores, such as ibuprofen, naproxen, and aspirin, may help lessen physical symptoms, such as cramps, headaches, backaches, and breast tenderness. Some women find that taking an over-the-counter pain reliever right before their period lessens the amount of pain and bleeding they experience during their period. Do keep in mind, though, that nonsteroidal anti-inflammatory drugs (NSAIDs) sometimes come with significant side effects to your kidneys and liver.

Midol

Many women take Midol for PMS. You should be aware that Midol is acetaminophen combined with a diuretic and caffeine. First, it is important to know that acetaminophen has been known to cause serious liver damage in larger doses—so much so that the packaging now includes a black-box warning that says:

> Severe liver damage may occur if
>
> - an adult takes more than 4,000 milligrams of acetaminophen in twenty-four hours (**that is just eight pills over twenty-four hours**).
>
> - an adult has three or more alcoholic drinks every day while using this product.

Both of which are what many people do when they have really, really bad cramps. Second, caffeine has been shown to increase premenstrual breast tenderness, and bloating—for which the diuretic is added—is only one of twelve symptoms associated with PMS, so overall Midol is an imperfect solution.

TENS Units

A new female-focused company is making TENS units to manage period pain. TENS units, which send electrical pulses through the skin in order to disrupt pain signals, have been used for a while now for managing pain, and they can be really useful for getting some short-term relief. But they won't help you understand the underlying issues or think about how to "fix" them.

CBD-Infused Tampons and Suppositories

So I tried both the tampon and the suppository, which is a little waxy ball with a dose of cannabidiol (CBD) and/or tetrahydrocannabinol (THC), either of which may be illegal depending upon where you live. I tried them mostly out of curiosity and because it was a great idea to make having your period a little more fun. While some consumers are reporting the suppository and the tampon can decrease your pain temporarily, there is very little research supporting the use of CBD or THC for menstrual pain relief. The main problem is that in order to keep the suppository in place long enough to work, you have to pretty much lie down. I don't know about you, but this girl has too much shit to do to lie down and get a little high every time her period comes. I didn't feel much relief from the tampon, but I don't have very much cramping in the first place.

Vitamins

There are a few options for supplements that are designed for women's health and PMS. Generally speaking, they are pretty useful if your diet isn't what it should be. Look, in order to have a good period, you need adequate calcium, magnesium, and vitamin B12. I prefer to get these nutrients from food rather than vitamins because absorption from the latter is typically inferior, as is the quality of the nutrients in a synthesized form. But if you have a significant nutrient deficiency and experience terrible cramps, they can be useful. If not, you can expect a 15 to 20 percent change in your symptoms. And taking supplements is still no way to get to all the roots of the problem.

Seed Cycling

One of my friends and colleagues, as well as a number of other clinicians, is starting to use food more and more prescriptively. I don't have a ton of experience with seed cycling, but I wanted to include it here because it's a new trend that's producing some positive results, especially for women who aren't getting their periods. So I asked Nicole Jardim, a certified women's health coach and the author of *The Happy Balance: The Original Plant-Based Approach for Hormone Health* and the forthcoming *Fix Your Period: Banish Bloating, Conquer Cramps, Manage Moodiness, and Become a Menstruation Maven* to explain seed cycling for us. Here's what she said:

> Seed cycling is a technique in which you rotate four different types of seeds according to which phase of

the menstrual cycle you are in. These seeds include pumpkin, flax, sesame, and sunflower seeds. This combination of seeds contains a wide variety of vitamins, minerals, and essential fatty acids that help support ovarian hormone production (think estrogen and progesterone) and thus overall menstrual health. Some of these include magnesium, zinc, iron, copper, and calcium. And let's not forget fiber, which will support the body's elimination of used-up estrogen! Seed cycling works well for women with irregular or missing periods, anovulatory cycles, and painful periods, as well as for women with a short luteal phase [short cycles] and heavy periods.

Here is how you do it. In the first half of your cycle, known as the follicular phase, from days 1 to 14, eat a tablespoon each of pumpkin seeds and ground flaxseeds every day. If you do not have a period, start day 1 of seed cycling on the first day of the new moon.

In the second half of your cycle, known as the luteal phase, from days 15 to 28, eat a tablespoon each of sunflower and sesame seeds. For women with regular cycles between twenty-five and thirty-five days long who don't ovulate on day 14, take the first round of seeds until you ovulate and switch to phase 2 seeds the day after you ovulate.

For women with irregular periods, long cycles, or missing periods, switch back to day 1 seeds on day 29. Once you get your period, start over with day 1 seeds and continue according to the above instructions. Flaxseeds should always be ground rather than consumed whole, and all of your seeds should be stored in the fridge to keep them from going rancid.

Herbal Supplements

I know we already discussed vitamins, but here I mean clinical-grade, plant-based herbal supplements. There are good data on the use of traditional Chinese medicine for managing the symptoms of PMS, PMDD, and menstrual cramping. In one study for PMDD, the most severe kind of PMS, the base formula we settled on was effective for more than 75 percent of women, with 46.7 percent of women achieving remission according to the Hamilton Depression Rating Scale (HAM-D) depression rating scale. Eighty-one percent of patients at the conclusion of the study no longer met the DSM-IV criteria for PMDD. For cramps, an industry-leading Cochrane Systematic Review of thirty-nine randomized control trials, including more than 3,400 women, found that herbal formulas like ours were almost twice as effective for treating menstrual pain as pharmaceutical treatments like over-the-counter painkillers or birth control pills, all without significant adverse effects.

They work well because they are typically not attempting to override a symptom but actually correct some of the underlying issues that cause the symptom in the first place. Remember, this is the physiological function from the traditional Chinese medicine point of view, so some of these explanations may seem different from conventional reproductive pathophysiology. In order to have optimized periods, a few organ systems have to be functioning well. First, there must be enough metabolic activity (and heat) in order to take the food you are consuming, separate the nutrients, convert it into energy, and use those nutrients and energy to make blood. When there is abundant blood, you will see adequate bleeding and hormonal metabolism by the liver. There are as many as forty symptoms associated with PMS and a variety of ways that menstrual cramping can present. It is virtually impossible to make a supplement to improve all of them. Instead, you have to combine the correct herbs that can improve and optimize the function of energy production, blood production, and hormone regulation. By using clinical-grade strength formulas, we are able to deliver potent solutions that are highly effective, while still being natural and safe for your body. This is a very different approach than using a supplement like magnesium or calcium to improve your cycle. Those are necessary micronutrients, but can easily be increased with food and only impact the symptoms when you in fact have a deficiency of those micronutrients that causes the problem in the first place.

Lifestyle and Behavior Modification

I'm not sure why, but modifiable lifestyle factors always get the short end of the stick, when in fact they can make enormous changes in cycle issues and, most important, they are free! The key is to know what the most important factors to start working on are, how to change them, and then how to modify your plan as you go so you continue to make progress. The next chapter outlines all the changes you can make and how to integrate them into your life.

Nothing

Bitching paired with a whole lot of nothing. My personal favorite (kidding). Sometimes folks just endure their situation, complain about it a heck of a lot, and hope that their periods will change. Maybe they will grow out of it. But sorry to be the bearer of bad news: cycle issues tend to get worse as you approach perimenopause. Since we don't really have any great solutions, I find that many women have just given up. They don't want to take birth control for the aforementioned reasons, they aren't into dealing with a shocking machine, and they don't think taking vitamins helps anything, so they suffer.

Understanding Your Ecosystem

In the last chapter, we covered all of the cycle factors that give us information about our overall health. We examined the length of our cycle, the timing of ovulation, the quality of our cervical discharge, the amount, intensity, and type of our PMS, the color and volume of our blood, the presence or absence of clotting, and our temperatures. And we learned how to interpret them as clues about how well our body is enjoying the way we're caring for it.

Here's the good news: you now have the information to understand the problems you've been seeing the good old American way—in isolation. You can see that you might have scanty bleeding or anxiety and insomnia with your PMS or that your cycle is less than twenty-eight days, which you now know is suboptimal. Most women, at some level, know all these pieces don't exist in a vacuum but rather are orchestrated into an interconnected system. We just don't know the way forward. Women ask me, "How can I fix my scanty period bleed? How can I extend my period from twenty-six to twenty-eight days to improve my fertility?"

There are certainly nutritional changes you can make and supplements you can take to improve your symptoms. I even built a company around some of those supplements because they work so well at managing symptoms. But I want something more for you. Not only do I want you to understand what's not optimal in your cycle and what that can tell you, but, more important, how all of the signs and symptoms plus your habits are inter-related. If you approach your health in this way, you'll see that it's actually a lot less work.

For example, you might have really bad PMS. Most women relate to their PMS as a crappy group of symptoms they have to deal with part of the month, but actually, all those shitty things are really symptoms of symptoms. *What?* I know, it isn't how we conventionally think about our issues, as being symptoms of something else, but let's look at how this plays out. So, you have PMS, but you also have really scanty bleeding. Well, if optimally women should have four days of bleeding and soak a tampon every four hours, one day of bleeding is a reflection of the fact that your ability to make abundant blood is not working well. Okay, we have to ask ourselves, where does blood come from? Blood is produced from our bone marrow. Hmmm, how is bone marrow produced?

Stay with me; this is why I developed algorithms to do this diagnostic work. Bone marrow is made of the building blocks of the food we eat. In order to build bone marrow effectively, two things need to be in place: you need to have abundant quality and quantity of nutrients in your diet, and your digestion—think back to high school biology—needs to be able to convert the food you are eating into energy and the exact nutrients needed to make bone marrow to make blood to support liver function to break down the hormones to keep you from having PMS.

If your digestion isn't functioning well, it's typically a symptom of something else to explore as well. What does digestion need to work well? It needs to have a healthy biome, be bug (parasite) free, encounter no foods that create sensitivities, and have enough heat. Wait, what does heat have to do with how well we turn food into energy? Think about it like this: you need heat to catalyze anything into energy. If you have a brand-new Maserati and the tank is full of high-performance, high-octane fuel but there's no spark plug, the car won't run. If the fuel isn't ignited, you are dead in the water. The same is true of your body. If your body temperature is really low, you have to struggle just to stay warm. You won't typically have a surplus of heat to catalyze the food you are eating into energy, which can leave you feeling fatigued despite the fact that you might be sleeping enough and eating an amazingly healthy diet. This is often the case for women who have low thyroid function (again, a symptom of a symptom) or even subclinical hypothyroidism (which means that your lab work looks normal but your symptoms look very similar to someone who has low thyroid function). So, you can see that what started off as one symptom took us down a virtual rabbit hole in which, after peeling back many layers of the onion, so to speak, we got to the root—which was either temperature regulation or digestive function.

Yes, it can be a little bit complicated to fit all the pieces together. But once you have a better understanding of how your signs and symptoms, cycle, and habits are all related, you can usually identify the issues that are contributing to the bigger problem in your ecosystem.

Let's take a look at a patient of mine named Kara (her name has been changed). She was thirty-two years old when she came to me with pretty significant PMS and menstrual cramping. She didn't really have a sense that anything else was wrong, apart from the fact that she became incredibly anxious and irritable before her period. Then when her period came, she had excruciating pain, every single month. When she discussed it with her doctor, he suggested she take four acetaminophen every four hours to manage the pain—and said he could start her on antidepressants for the mood swings. But Kara didn't like the idea of taking too much acetaminophen every single month, especially given the black-box warning, and putting her liver at risk. She didn't feel as though she was clinically depressed, so she wasn't into the idea of taking antidepressants, but her PMS was really bad in terms of mood swings and bloating. The way her cycle was going every single month was really impacting her life, her relationships, and her general ability to bring her best to the table.

Kara admitted that she was also quite tired every day but pushed through with willpower and caffeine. At night she had a hard time falling asleep and woke up often throughout the night. She also felt cold all the time. Her period brought two days of really heavy bleeding, soaking a tampon every hour, with tremendous pain and clotting. The blood was dark, and even when she took the acetaminophen it didn't make the pain go away; it just made it manageable. After two days the blood became pink and watery, and she could go a whole day without changing even a light pad.

After we talked about her signs and symptoms, I asked her about her habits: what does she eat, how does she manage stress, does she exercise, and if so, how much, what kind, and how often?

Here's our Q&A.

KIRSTEN: What do you eat?

KARA: I have a really healthy diet.

KIRSTEN: Can you give me a sense of what your average breakfast, lunch, dinner, and snacks are?

KARA: Sure. For breakfast I usually have a smoothie.

KIRSTEN: Okay, what's in it?

KARA: Oh, lots of good stuff like apple juice, blueberries, and half a banana. And some protein powder.

KIRSTEN: Yeah, there are a lot of healthy foods in that, except maybe it seems like a heck of a lot of sugar to start the day. Tell me about lunch.

KARA: I'm often on the go, so I will typically grab a protein bar or a salad.

KIRSTEN: Okay, tell me about your salad. What kind of ingredients do you like to put in your salad?

KARA: I like to keep it pretty simple, with iceberg lettuce because it's so crunchy, some sliced cucumbers and tomatoes, and some healthy ranch dressing.

KIRSTEN: [Thinking: Okay, on the surface this looks good, but your body needs a wide variety of nutrient-rich foods like broccoli, kale, organic animal products, nuts, and avocados. Here we have the bar made largely of synthesized proteins, and her salad has minimal nutritional value.] Okay, I can see you are really making a good effort to healthily feed yourself. Let's look at what else you are eating. How about dinner?

KARA: Since I eat so healthfully during the day, I usually splurge at dinner. I might have veggie pizza or Chinese takeout.

KIRSTEN: Oh, actually, those are pretty good choices if you are eating out. What about snacks?

KARA: I don't really snack very much. I'm pretty satisfied having a caramel macchiato in the afternoon to boost my energy.

KIRSTEN: [Thinking: Dang, okay, we have a bit of work to do.] Seems like you have a pretty stressful job. How do you cope with your stress?

KARA: I work out like crazy. It is the only thing that saves me. Well . . . and a few glasses of wine after work.

KIRSTEN: Gotcha. Tell me more about your workouts. How long, and what do you do?

KARA: I work out pretty much every day. Sometimes I work out twice a day. I usually do a ninety-minute spin class or CrossFit.

KIRSTEN: That's sweaty work! So, do you think you feel more cold or hot compared to other people?

KARA: I'm so cold all the time. I even wear a sweater in the summer when I'm inside. I don't know why they need to put the air on *so* cold in Texas.

As we discussed earlier, we have to keep asking ourselves what larger issues our symptoms are side effects of. And we have to keep examining our habits to see where we might be working against ourselves. From Kara's case study, we can see that she had pretty significant PMS, cramping, heavy then scanty bleeding, fatigue, and cold. Her body was exhausted and wasn't making much blood. That was probably impacting her liver's ability to break down hormones at the end of her cycle and to regulate the flow of blood, which was contributing to her cramping. If we look at her digestion, we can see that although she *thought* her diet was pretty healthy, it lacked adequate nutrients, which was leaving her feeling drained. Despite the fact that she was really tired all the time, she insisted on working out a ton. She believed that if she worked out more and harder, she would get fitter and alleviate her fatigue. That couldn't be further from the truth. If your tank is empty, what you need is rest. I typically tell patients that strenuous workouts are reserved for folks who have sustainable energy levels above 7 or 8 out of 10. Otherwise, moderate exercise such as walking, swimming, and yoga are the way to go.

If you're working on improving and optimizing your health, you have to listen to what your body needs in order to get better. Remember that exercising, though incredibly good for you and essential for good health, comes in many forms and overdoing it can really compromise your blood. When you exercise, you are contracting your muscles powerfully. Each time you do so, your body uses oxygen and nutrients to keep working. The harder you work, the bigger the demand. Guess what the mechanism is for delivering those nutrients? You got it, your blood.

But back to Kara. You can see that she was eating a lot of salads and feeling really cold. Because her metabolic activity was so low, she wasn't able to digest her food well enough to convert it into energy. Her diet was okay, but she couldn't seem to get any juice out of it. Since she wasn't getting sufficient nourishment out of her food, her ability to break down food, convert it into energy, and then extract the building blocks needed to make bone marrow and then blood production was impaired. When this happens, a lot of PMS symptoms occur.

In order to help Kara get better, I suggested a few things:

1. First, she needed to significantly reduce the intensity and frequency of her workouts so she could recover her resources of energy and blood.

2. Next, she needed to reduce the amount of sugar in her diet and increase the amount of nutrient-rich foods (clean animal products and tons of vegetables). Ideally, she would also include more warming foods, such as ginger, cinnamon, garlic, and turmeric, to fire up her metabolism and iron-rich foods to help her make more blood.

3. She needed to prioritize sleep and learn strategies to manage stress such as meditation or breathing exercises.

4. Finally, she should supplement her diet with herbs to improve her liver function while her body is recovering.

Instead of focusing on her one symptom of PMS or cramping, we looked at her whole ecosystem of signs, symptoms, and habits and customized a combination of rest, high-quality and precise nutritional interventions, and herbs. The added benefit of approaching your health in this way is that not only will the original complaints get better, but so will your overall health.

Take Action!

Want to know more about your cycle? You can go to www.Foreverbrazen and take the quiz to get a personalized report on your cycle.

6

········

HOW TO BIOHACK
YOUR PERIOD, PART 2

Lifestyle Changes

*Systems thinking is a discipline for seeing wholes. It is a
framework for seeing interrelationships rather than things, for
seeing "patterns of change" rather than static "snapshots."*

— PETER SENGE

love this quote because although Senge was applying it to
business, we can easily translate it to our health. Everything is
intertwined with everything else.

I've talked about how in our Western worldview, we have the
tendency to see everything in isolation, not as part of a whole
organic system. A consequence of that view is to look at each of
your habits as an individual aspect of your lifestyle. It can be difficult to imagine how your mind-set is related to your exercise
routine or how your sleep could have any impact on what you eat.
Because of this limited point of view, all of us have been trained to

be very myopic in our perspective on what's possible in our lives. The result is incredibly frustrating. When you try to change one habit without looking at all of them together as an interdependent system, it's difficult to feel as though you're making progress.

So, sure, it can take effort to get past focusing on an individual behavior—such as not drinking enough water or snacking too much after dinner—and to see how all your habits interact to reinforce or undermine one another. The good news is that once you do see the whole matrix of interconnected habits, you begin to realize if you make small positive behavior changes in one area, it becomes easier to make additional changes in other areas. One little change enables another and then another, and suddenly you've made incremental changes in several areas and they're now producing significant changes in the whole giant ecosystem that is you.

Before we get into the nitty-gritty, though, I want to point out something that's working against all of us in our attempts to be healthy. In a culture like ours, which values being a badass, it means you have to do more, work harder, work longer, ignore your body, and, yes, sleep less than everyone else. Even if that's not you (but I bet it is), it sounds familiar, right? This mind-set is extremely pervasive. We believe strongly that more is more in practically every situation.

Here's a great example. In my clinic, I use infrared heating lamps that I shine on my patients' abdomens to raise their internal temperature. These suckers get really, really hot, and of course I tell patients to move the lamp if it gets uncomfortable. One day I went into the treatment room at the end of a session and noticed that the patient's stomach was blazing red. Shocked and frankly concerned that we had burned her, I moved the lamp and asked, "Oh, gosh, wasn't that hurting you? Why didn't you ring the bell so I could come and adjust it for you?" She said, "Well, I know you want to raise my temperature, so I figured if warm was good, blazing hot was better." I said, "But it had to feel like it was burning your skin, no?" And she said, "I didn't care. I'm tough, and I can endure anything."

Frankly, it made me sad to hear that. It wasn't the first time a patient had told me that she was willing to endure anything to get ahead. This mentality can serve us when we use it in a balanced way that doesn't hurt our bodies, minds, or overall health. But often, we use our fortitude in the wrong way (and women are about as badass as they come even when their periods are kicking their butts). The problem is that this mind-set has shifted away from being positive and useful and been transformed into a pathology that's actually hurting many of us. We'll work and work and work to achieve our goals and dreams, but for so many of us, all that work comes at the cost of both our physical and our mental health. That misdirected overachiever mind-set is taxing our bodies and minds and significantly impacting our health, cycles, and ability to reproduce.

I have had many teachers who helped deepen my understanding of this mind-set, how it worked against me (and my patients), and how to channel it more productively. One of them was my brilliant and sage midwife, Laurie Fremgen.

Having a midwife deliver your children at home is a very different experience from having a hospital birth. Obviously, you don't get an epidural, so while your baby is growing inside you, you spend quite a lot of time with the midwife, preparing for the experience. I could wax romantic ad nauseum about how much I loved my birth experience, but I will save that for my book on pregnancy and fertility. For now, here's an insight Laurie gave me that I think will help you.

No more than ten minutes into my first conversation with Laurie, she said, "You know, Kirsten, the only way to get a baby out is to surrender."

"I've never surrendered to anything in my life. I'm the feistiest, most firecracker, hardest-working unstoppable bitch out there. I don't surrender to anything. It isn't in my DNA," I told her. (You can see my mind-set in action.)

"I know," she said. "I figured as much."

"Laurie, do you think I'm a control freak?" I asked.

"Well, I think if you could control the weather you probably would."

Shit.

Then she said something so powerful that it changed me forever. She said, "Look, it's clear to me that you're a producer. You can get shit done. You can use your will to make things happen. But you're just using it to control and drive outcomes. I want to ask you to begin to use your power for something else. I want you to use your will to force yourself to become a black belt in surrender. Just like you trained to be an athlete all your life, now use those skills to train yourself in surrender. Every time your mother-in-law [who, by the way, I actually adore, but Laurie didn't know that] tries to dominate you, surrender, let her do it. Encourage her to do it. When you're in traffic and jerks are trying to cut in front of you, surrender. Smile at them, let them in, and have gratitude for another swing at the plate of surrender practice. The more you practice, the easier it will be for you to surrender anytime you want. When you feel the pull of the desire to overwork, to compete, to dominate, surrender, if even just for a few minutes or hours. And as you do, the hook of control will start to dissolve, and you'll actually start to get access to real power instead of the perceived power of control. Remember, the greatest power doesn't come from control and domination. It comes from the ability to let go of anything at any time. When you're a black belt at surrender, nothing and no one can control you."

Holy crap! I wanted that. So I used my pregnancy as an opportunity to learn how to transform my relationship with control, drive, and overwork.

I encourage you, too, to start practicing surrendering a little bit every day. See what it feels like to let go. Can you find some freedom? A little more breath in your lungs? A little more ease in your heart? If you can keep practicing this, it will help you start making behavior changes faster and more easily, and your life will be more joyful. The more you are able to do this, the easier behavior and habit change will be for you.

● ● ●

Before we delve into each habit, I want to talk about using the phases of your cycle to make your changes more precisely and amplify the benefits you get from them. The easiest way to understand this is to break your cycle into three phases: bleeding, follicular, and luteal.

MENSTRUAL CYCLE

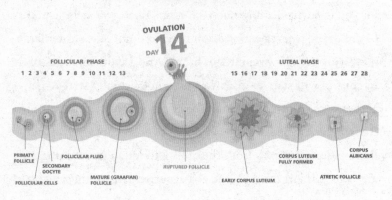

Then we'll identify where each of your symptoms falls in your cycle. This will help you determine how to change your habits, including nutrition, sleeping, and exercise, accordingly and help you improve those things.

For example, often patients come into my office all inspired and announce that they started a cleanse on January 1 (when it's freezing out, even in Texas). This makes no sense, when you stop to think that winter is the time when we naturally tend to accumulate fat to help our bodies fare better in extreme cold temperatures. We typically eat a little more and gain a bit of additional weight. We sleep more (even if we can't actually hibernate), and the increased nutrition and rest can actually be restorative. Our natural inclination at this time of year isn't to purge and reduce, it's to slow down and store—and be restored. In spring, by contrast, all of our energy is alive. The things that were dead or hibernating in the winter revive or wake up, and we all begin to shed what we no longer need. Now the body is ready for some pruning to discard whatever's no longer necessary. Doing a cleanse in springtime makes perfect sense.

In each phase of your cycle, there are changes that will work better with your natural tendencies, depending on which of the three phases you're in. Each phase has a specific function, and when your body is performing that function, that phase can be your amplifier to make changes in your health and cycle faster and more efficiently.

I want to define a term that every person with a period should know because it's an important term to be able to talk about, track, and regulate your cycle: *cycle day 1*. This is a critical data point for every woman with a period. Cycle day 1 is the first day of real bleeding and helps us benchmark the rest of the cycle for a variety of applications, from predicting ovulation and your period to knowing the best days to do certain hormonal blood tests.

Now let's take a deep dive into the phases.

- **Bleeding** (cycle days 1 to 4). Conventionally, this is still part of the follicular phase, but I divide them because from a therapeutic perspective, we want to accomplish different things in each phase according to your body's natural inclination. Essentially, this is the phase when you are discharging the unused uterine lining if you aren't pregnant. Your body's natural inclination is to discharge what isn't necessary. Using food, exercise, and the right Chinese herbs can make a huge difference in the color, quality, and quantity of your menstrual blood and the amount of pain you experience each month.

- **Follicular phase** (cycle days 4 to 14). This is called the follicular phase because of the increasing amounts of follicle-stimulating hormone (FSH) produced by your body during this phase. FSH helps develop the follicles in the ovary, which will ultimately release an egg during ovulation several weeks later. After about six days of your follicular phase, your estrogen levels rise to help thicken your uterine lining, onto which the egg will implant itself if fertilization occurs. This is the time when things are accumulating and building. If we follow the body's natural inclination, this is when we want to focus on energy and blood production.

- **Ovulation** (cycle day 14). This is not a phase; I just want to remind you that your mature egg has left the ovary and is ready to be fertilized!

- **Luteal phase** (cycle days 15 to 28). Okay, so you ovulated. Now what? Now the little sac that held your egg, called the corpus luteum, has collapsed and begins to produce progesterone. The progesterone works to help thicken your uterine lining in case there is a fertilized egg ready to implant itself. If implantation doesn't occur in the next ten to fifteen days, your body will eliminate the lining by starting your period in conjunction with a drop in your progesterone level.

Healthy habits form the foundation on which your periods can flourish during each step of your cycle. Now let's examine how each of the below factors affects your health, cycle, and fertility individually—and how you can develop habits to support a healthier menstrual cycle.

- Sleep

- Exercise

- Nutrition

- Mind-set

- Stress management

- Hydration

- Supplements

- Community support and connection

Sleep

I am a little fanatical about sleep. Pretty much no matter what you do, if you can't fall asleep, stay asleep, and wake up rested, it's incredibly difficult to fix anything else. I'm not saying it's impossible, but improper sleep is a huge roadblock to getting better. Without enough sleep, your decision-making skills diminish, your response time slows, and your risk of developing stroke, cancer, and heart disease increases. New research shows that operating on too little sleep is roughly equivalent to being legally drunk.[1]

Though an hour of sleep missed here or there doesn't seem like a huge deal, when you compound the effects over time, they can be massive. Sleep deficit doesn't just go away, so missing an hour a night is like pulling an all-nighter once a week! The amount of shut-eye you get per night is especially significant to your reproductive ability. Hormonal signals that control a number of reproductive functions are regulated during sleep, so even though you may think you're just missing extra "beauty" sleep, you may actually be contributing to your period problems.

Let's learn a little bit about these hormones.

- **Leptin.** Though progesterone, estrogen, luteinizing hormone, and follicle-stimulating hormone are all affected by your sleep patterns, one of the most important hormones altered by sleep pattern is leptin. Leptin is essential for promoting ovulation and regulating menstruation. In addition, it increases the weight of the uterus—and that increase in weight is an indication that the lining is ideal for embryo implantation. When your sleep is interrupted, your leptin level drops, causing disruption in your menstrual cycles, irregular ovulation, and a scanty uterine lining. Leptin is also really important because it influences your levels of appetite and weight gain. When you are not sleeping well, your leptin levels can decline, making you hungrier and more likely to gain weight. Who wants that?

- **Cortisol.** Sleep also has an impact on cortisol function. When you're not sleeping enough, your body makes up for the resulting lack of energy by producing more of the stress hormone cortisol to power you through the day. An increase in cortisol caused by sleep deprivation not only taxes your adrenal glands but has a hugely negative impact on progesterone levels as well. Progesterone is recruited to produce increased cortisol, taking it away from its important fertility-related tasks such as preparing the endometrium for implantation and maintaining early pregnancy. Remember, even if you are not trying to get pregnant, your optimal health will be ultimately demonstrated by your fertility.

- **Insulin.** Adequate sleep is also required to maintain a healthy metabolism. In a study of healthy college students, researchers found that participants whose sleep was repeatedly disturbed, even for one night, were found to exhibit decreased sensitivity to insulin, a condition that is generally a warning sign of type 2 diabetes. When your body doesn't get the sleep it needs, it revs up your desire for calories to keep it running. Your appetite increases, and this can cause weight gain, which has been associated with ovulatory irregularity and decreased fertility. You also increase your risk for metabolic diseases such as type 2 diabetes and PCOS.[2]

Your body, especially the reproductive system, is controlled by a complex hormone system—a system that starts to break down if you don't get enough sleep. Without proper sleep, our bodies and our reproductive systems begin to shut down. Sleep experts agree that improving your sleep hygiene—your sleeping environment and habits—is the most important step to restoring normal, healthy sleep.

Exercise

Most of the patients I've worked with over the last twenty years have told me they needed to exercise more. Some of them were working out daily and some even twice a day. People talk about the menstrual cycle being a curse, but I actually think the unachievable perfect body is a much more devastating curse for women and their health. I see the hundreds of thousands of Instagram followers of the women who are chronicling their physical transformations from what I would call pretty nice bodies to super jacked divas. Don't get me wrong, I follow them, too. They are inspiring as hell, and I want to look like that in a thong bikini, too. The problem is that I've treated many women who look like this, and although they look super healthy on the outside, when I ask them about their periods, they look at me with surprise, as if to ask, "What does that have to do with anything?" Then they proceed to tell me that their periods are shit storms with only a little bleeding, lots of cramping, clotting, irregular cycles, and so on. We've been lured into believing that "jacked" means super healthy, but if we're using our menstrual cycles as barometers of our health, jacked has nothing to do with it. In fact, oftentimes it can give women a false sense of confidence in their health because of how their bodies look on the outside.

In our culture, it's considered an immutable fact of nature that the more you work out, the healthier you are, and that exercising more, even if you're tired, is good for you. You're probably even nodding your head in agreement with those statements, thinking "Well, that's true." Remember a page or two ago, where we spoke about control and surrender? I'm going to ask you to start practicing letting go of your current belief system and to stay with me here. This idea is one that most people really want to resist, but hang in there, I'll get you to the finish line.

First, yes, exercise is essential to your cycle, your health, and your well-being. That we agree on! However, your body's current needs should dictate the kind of exercise you do and the frequency and duration of your workouts; as you get healthier, you should modify your workouts accordingly on an ongoing basis.

As you think about creating the ideal workout for you right now, the first question to ask yourself is this: on a scale of 1 to 10 (1 being you can't get out of bed much and 10 meaning not maniacally energetic but just that you have solid energy all day), what is your energy level like without any caffeine? (Note: You may have to give up caffeine for a few days to know what your actual energy level is.) Few women I have met have energy levels above 8 in a sustainable way without any caffeine. Most fall somewhere between 5 and 7, but a significant proportion of them are below 5. In my experience most women are pretty exhausted.

If you're exhausted (below 5), it's possible that you're running on pure adrenaline. People who've gotten to that point report having high levels of energy, and when they start to get more rest, they actually feel more tired at first. Weird, right? Not really. What's happening is that when you get really exhausted, your body's only fuel source is adrenaline. When you stop driving so hard and start resting, the mechanism that was pumping adrenaline into your system to basically keep you alive starts slowing down because your body believes the crisis is going away. Without the massive continuous adrenaline dump, you start experiencing your actual energy level, which is exhausted. So at least for a while, the more an exhausted person rests and sleeps, the more tired she feels. Interestingly, someone in this situation may want to exercise, because that will produce an adrenaline/endorphin dump that temporarily feels like an improvement.

But let's assume that you're not *that* exhausted. If your energy is below 7, I wouldn't suggest doing any intense workouts such as spinning or CrossFit because there's no surplus of energy for you to burn through. You may think that if you work out harder, you'll make more energy. And yes, a big workout will leave you feeling temporarily energized because of the boost in endorphins, but you'll have emptied your tank just a little more.

And let's face it: better health and even feeling good aren't our only motivations for exercising. We also work out to improve the appearance of our bodies. But even here moderation is the way to go. When you're exhausted, you're producing a lot of adrenaline, which converts to cortisol, which in turn contributes to belly fat—the same damn thing we're doing a million crunches a day to get rid of.

So what to do?

Again, even for exhausted individuals, I'm not suggesting no exercise at all. I'm suggesting a high degree of moderation: paring down your workouts to thirty minutes or less every day, doing activities such as walking (not power walking, just good old brisk walking), hatha yoga (less intense than ashtanga yoga, with longer poses and deeper breath work), restorative yoga (the most effective), and tai chi. People often think that tai chi isn't really a form of exercise but a kind of meditation old Chinese people do in parks. That couldn't be further from the truth! An interesting thing happened when a group of researchers were looking to validate the notion that regular cardiovascular exercise (such as brisk walking or jogging) for approximately five to six hours a week would reduce the morbidity caused by cardiovascular events. The researchers included tai chi as one of the interventions. I suspect that they thought it would have no effect and act as a "control." What happened next surprised everyone. The researchers found that the tai chi group had reduced their morbidity risk as much as the individuals who were jogging or brisk walking. The study demonstrated that we don't have to kill ourselves working out to have a significant impact on heart health. So my point is, don't stop exercising—just look for ways to move your body and improve blood flow that won't further exhaust you until your energy level is at least a solid 7.

Nutrition

There are so many theories about how and what to eat—from intermittent fasting to veganism to ketogenic. All of these different approaches have data to support their health benefits. There are books out there telling you what you should eat to regulate your cycle. What I want you to know is that no one way of eating is right for everyone. You have to continue to look at your body as an ecosystem and find the nutrition that will support you as you work with all of your specific issues. And you'll want to modify your diet to adjust to your body's changing needs. If we get even more granular, each phase of your cycle will respond to different types of food as well.

Let me give you an example. One patient who happened to be a vegan came to me for her severe PMS. She thought she was really healthy otherwise. Every month, however, as soon as she ovulated, her breasts would get really sore, she would experience extreme anxiety, and her sleep would be really disturbed by waking up every few hours. She had been having these experiences since she got her period but since she turned thirty-five, everything seemed to be getting a lot worse. Remember, despite all of this, she said she was really healthy. When I asked about her period she said she was lucky because there was hardly any blood at all. She typically had just one day of bleeding with heavy clotting and pain, and then a few days of rusty spotting. Earlier I mentioned that ideally you want four days of your blood soaking a tampon or pad every four hours? That's four days, not more or less. In my experience, the fewer days of bleeding the more PMS symptoms I saw and with more symptoms like anxiety vs. rage/irritability. In order to improve her PMS, we needed to make more blood to help her liver metabolize the excess hormones at the end of her cycle. The obvious solution would be to increase her intake of iron-rich foods. That makes perfect sense, right? Wrong. First, if you are a vegan, this is challenging to do from only veggies and without any naturally occurring vitamin B12 in your diet. Second, if I had her start pounding iron-rich foods and make a bunch of new blood, we would have actually made more clotting and more pain. Yikes, wrong direction. First you have to address the cause of the clotting and use herbs to dissolve the clots, and then you can start building up your blood. Be sure to consult a qualified herbalist to help, or you can try Brazen Cramp Support to get started.

Remember, something different is happening in each of your cycle's phases, and different people have different problems during each one. So if you eat the same thing all the time, you miss the opportunity to use food as medicine, to customize and curate the way you eat in response to the season and the environment. Eating a variety of foods during each phase of the menstrual cycle can make a significant difference in your health. There's certainly a science to doing this, but don't worry, in the next chapter, I'm going to break it down into very simple starting points so you can begin working on customizing the way you eat—depending on your closest archetype.

Mind-set

Did you know that how you think is a kind of habit? On the most superficial level, some people are more optimistic (as opposed to pessimistic). I land on the side of optimism, so much so that one of my friends used to tell me that I had pathological optimism. I so believe that only good can come to me that sometimes I struggle to forecast potential problems and make plans to prevent them. Even though optimism is typically viewed as something positive, you can see how it can be taken to an extreme. What about you? Do you see the glass as half full or half empty?

When you've been sick for a long time, especially when you've had something that we've been taught to just ignore, it can be very easy to view yourself as someone who just isn't good, powerful, or healthy when it comes to issues related to your period.

When my MS was really active and I could hardly walk without a cane, I was always scared that something was going to trigger my body to rebel against me and make some other part of my body stop working. I constantly worried I would wake up blind, because when I refused to take the medication my doctors had suggested, they always said, "Okay, I hope you don't wake up blind." I allowed that comment to determine my mind-set. I believed that I was destined for a wheelchair because I couldn't see any way out of it. I am guessing that many of you have a similar kind of mind-set. When there are no obvious solutions to your problems, it's very natural for your mind to create a story called "This Shit Is Hopeless, So Just Try to Survive."

What exactly is your mind-set? It's what you believe to be true; what you allow your mind to tell you that you then literally live into reality. Until you can identify your mind-set, everything else in this book won't be as powerful.

If you think you're sick, if you think your periods are normal even though you're suffering, if you think you're a wimp because you're complaining about pain, if you think you have no way out, you don't.

Your mind cannot tell the difference between what you're imagining and reality. When you think, you use your imagination to make up stories about yourself.

Here are just a few I hear often:

- I am fat.

- I am stupid.

- I am ugly.

- I am worthless.

- I am not enough.

- I am sick.

- I have endometriosis.

- I feel crazy.

Yes, all of those are stories that are based upon your interpretation of facts. Let's take a few of these that I hear most often and then look at the facts.

"I am fat." "I weigh 135 pounds and am five foot three" suddenly becomes "I am fat." The only true thing is that I weigh 135 pounds and am five foot three. Then I created a story that because of those facts, I am fat. Fat is just a story.

"I am stupid." I make a mistake almost every time I book a flight, often missing flights or showing up at the airport at the wrong time (true). I created a story that because of those things, I am stupid. I ignore the other facts: I own a bunch of patents, have published papers in scholarly journals, have won awards, and so on. Yet when I miss a flight, I feel like an idiot and it erases every other piece of data that supports the fact that I am not stupid at all.

"I am sick." You may have a diagnosable disease such as endometriosis or PCOS, infertility, diabetes, or even cancer, or you may have a cluster of symptoms no one can figure out; you just don't feel well most days. But there is a huge difference between that and the mind-set "I am sick." Today I have low energy. I have pain in my abdomen. My head is hurting. Those are the facts. Beyond that is a story that means something about who you are at the core. If we believe that what we tell ourselves is reality, having a mind-set of "I am sick" will put us into a situation in which our mind is constantly reinforcing and actively looking for evidence to support that story. Remember that you will see what you look for, and if you are looking, consciously or unconsciously, for evidence that you are sick, you will most certainly find it. It's so easy to believe that the things we tell ourselves are true. But if you can stay with just the facts, ma'am, you can begin to set yourself free.

> *Where the mind goes the body follows.*
> —HUANG DI NEI JING

When I was trying to recover my health after my MS diagnosis, I was intensively studying mind-set and the impact it has on our health. I was so persuaded by the data that I made a conscious decision not to say I had MS anymore. In fact, only in writing this book have I even talked about my health in terms of my previous diagnosis.

Simply not saying I had MS didn't make my MS go into remission, obviously, but I was interested in disentangling my mind from the idea that I had MS. When I had neurological problems, instead of saying "Oh, that's from my MS," I started saying "I feel tired today" or "My arm is weaker than usual" or "I am falling a lot today." I tried to keep the description to things that were as factual as possible and avoid extrapolating those facts to a story.

I love mind-set work for several reasons. First, I do believe it's more powerful than anything else I can teach you in this book. Second, it's free. Third, it's one of the few things that both exponentially improves the quality of your life and gives you agency where you never had it before. You don't need any special tools or gadgets. All you have to do is listen to what you are allowing your mind to tell you. Start looking at your mind like an outsider, and choose whether or not to listen to the inner voice telling those stories, and you'll start to liberate yourself from constraints—and that is when massive healing can start to happen. Plus freedom is almost always more fun than being a prisoner of your mind, right?

So today, I want you to start listening to the stories you have been creating about what is possible for your health, your career, your finances, your relationships, and whatever else you spend time thinking about. Ask yourself: are these the stories I want to be exposing myself to on a daily basis? You don't have to do anything else today or even this week. Just listen. Bonus points if you share them with a girlfriend and have a good laugh about how silly and restrictive they are. Remember, they're just stories. Don't give them more power than they deserve.

After you have spent a few weeks getting acquainted with your not-so-helpful, constantly prattling mind, make a list of the main conversations you want to eliminate because they're no longer useful in your pursuit of general badassery and optimal health. Now the fun part begins. Start creating *new* stories about what's possible. Why not make up a story that you'd be excited to live in? Play big, break things with your mind, do the impossible, be impossible, and be hypervigilant about continuing to eliminate the stories that limit and hurt you and blow up the stories that will set you free.

Stress Management

Now that you're making friends with your mind, you're ready to take on another habit: dealing effectively with stress. Stress is a curious thing: pretty much everybody has a fair amount of it, but there are wide differences in how well our bodies are able to tolerate it. Some patients I've worked with have been under extreme pressure and stress and their bodies have seemed relatively resilient to it, whereas others have had what I would describe as pretty moderate stress, and it was practically killing them. For example, I had a patient who was working about a hundred hours a week trying to become a partner in a law firm. She was so passionate about the law and her work that spending so many taxing hours working had very little effect on her body. She got so much joy from her work that it fed and supported her mind and body. On the other hand, I had a patient who was working very moderately with moderate amounts of stress, but the impact on her adrenal glands and reproductive system was huge. There are no data to support this, but I have a theory that it actually relates to how introverted versus extroverted a person is. We know that the more introverted you are, the more sensitive your nervous system is to your environment. Conversely, the more extroverted you are, the more your body responds positively to a lot of stimuli. I think this may also dictate how our body responds to intense work and stress. Again, that's just a theory.

To understand the impact of stress, let's break it down into two main types. There's good stress (yes, that is a thing), and there's chronic stress, which is terrible for your health.

First, let's look at a good stress response. Our bodies want to do whatever will help us be healthy. Reacting powerfully to stressful circumstances is an important survival mechanism for our species, and our bodies do it amazingly well. They are designed to react almost instantly with a flood of adrenaline to help us handle emergencies. When that happens, our fight-or-flight mechanism kicks in and we can suddenly have access to super-powers to either fight like crazy or run as fast as lightning. An evolutionary function that supports our survival, these tools can be incredibly effective—I'm sure you've seen videos of mothers doing things such as lifting cars off their children—but our bodies weren't designed to draw on our energy sources that way more than once in a while. When you're in fight-or-flight mode, adrenaline and cortisol flood your system, causing your blood pressure, breathing, and heart rate to increase so that you start feeling invincible. You need to fuel this beast, so a ton of glucose is released into your bloodstream for energy. Now, since you're in survival mode, your digestion, growth, and reproductive and immune system functions are suppressed, as well as the blood flow to your skin (although there are as yet no studies examining this, I would bet that uterine and ovarian blood flow is also decreased), and pain tolerance is increased. This is a very effective way for the body to deal with an emergency—occasionally. It's a beautiful ability to call up the necessary hormones and fuel to save your life and triage your organ function that conserves your energy until you're safe.

Unfortunately, most of us are so overworked, underfed, underslept, over- or underexercised, and feeling such tremendous pressure that instead of occasionally being in a state of good stress to survive a temporary struggle, we live in that state every day.

That's right, most of us are living in a state in which our nervous system is worried that we're about to die. Every day. That's how chronic, or bad, stress develops. Instead of thriving and creating every day, we exist in perpetual survival mode, and our bodies respond chemically in a way that over time can make us very sick. Instead of only ramping up to fight off an occasional bear attack, our nervous systems are going through the drill daily. Our bodies are flooded with adrenaline and cortisol (read: belly fat) and keep demanding glucose (insulin resistance, which interrupts ovulation) and slowing down digestion (weight gain, poor energy production, poor conversion of nutrients into blood for your cycle). This is happening every day, and it consumes so much of the precious resources our bodies need for good health. Given enough time, our adrenal glands are drained and it becomes more and more difficult to recover.

You might be worrying "Crap, I am really in trouble! I have a really stressful life and a lot of responsibility, and that simply isn't going to change. I'm screwed." Yes—but it's critically important to remember that being "stressed out" is also a mind-set. Research shows that our attitude toward stress deeply affects the impact that it can have on our bodies. Stanford University psychologist Kelly McGonigal has shown in her book *The Upside of Stress: Why Stress Is Good for You, and How to Get Good at It* that stress can make us stronger, smarter, and happier—if we learn how to open our minds to it.[3] Stanford Mind & Body Lab principal investigator Alia Crum showed that viewing stress as a helpful part of life, rather than harmful, is associated with better health, emotional well-being, and productivity at work—even during periods of high stress. How you think about stress— your mind-set—impacts how you cope with it.[4] For example, if you consider it a negative experience, you might cope with it by getting drunk or eating a giant slice of chocolate cake. Trying to avoid stress can make the situation worse. One study found that simply having the goal to avoid stress increased the long-term risk of outcomes such as depression, divorce, and getting fired by increasing people's reliance on harmful coping strategies. The good news is that when you can adjust your mind-set to see the stress in your life as something normal, something that cannot be avoided, it can even be helpful by encouraging better and more proactive coping strategies, such as figuring out a plan to tackle the source of the stress, looking to your friends or family for support, or looking for meaning through reflection or spiritual practices.

So how can you change your mind-set and relationship to your stress? McGonigal says that the three most protective beliefs about stress are:

1. To view your body's stress response as helpful, not debilitating—for example, to view stress as energy you can use.

2. To view yourself as able to handle, and even learn and grow from, the stress in your life.

3. To view stress as something that everyone deals with, not something that proves how uniquely screwed up you or your life is.

Hydration

Drinking water seems like a total no-brainer. Yes, we all know that we need to drink water, but most of us probably need to drink more than we do. Here are a few details about just how important water is for your health and your cycle.

Water accounts for about one-half to two-thirds of your weight. If you're at an appropriate weight, this is a good thing, but if you're overweight, it's more critical to pay attention to hydration because fat tissue has a lower percentage of water than lean tissue, making it more susceptible to dehydration and its serious impacts on the body and reproductive system.

Every cell, tissue, and organ in your body needs water to work properly. You need adequate hydration so your body can maintain its temperature, make cervical mucus, and protect your tissues, spinal cord, and joints. It also keeps sensitive areas, such as your eyes and your vagina, from feeling dry. You need to keep your body hydrated to retain optimum levels of moisture in those areas, as well as in your blood, bones, and brain.

Another reason water is so important is that it helps our bodies eliminate waste. Our bodies are designed to get rid of both liquid and solid waste, and without adequate hydration, the system stalls, leaving you constipated and loaded up with waste by-products. The kidneys, liver, and intestines all use water to help flush out waste. Adequate water intake enables your body to excrete waste through perspiration, urination, and defecation. If you're dehydrated, the liver can't function properly to clear waste and remove excess hormones that can contribute to hormonal imbalances.

Then there's digestion. Most people don't realize it, but digestion starts with your saliva, which is formed from, um, water. Your saliva contains enzymes that break down food and liquids, dissolve minerals and other nutrients, and then help convert those nutrients into blood, a substance that's also made up mostly of water. You also need water to break down soluble fiber, which keeps your poops (another mechanism of waste removal) in tip-top shape. There are a variety of suggestions about how much water is the right amount and countless studies supporting the various hypotheses. Keep it easy, and follow the eight-by-eight rule. That means try to drink eight 8-ounce glasses of water a day. You'll get the added benefit of increased metabolism (and who doesn't want that?) if you drink 17 ounces at one time. According to one study, participants' metabolic activity temporarily increased between 24 and 30 percent when they did so. The researchers also estimated that drinking 68 ounces (2 liters) in one day increases energy expenditure by about 96 calories.[5] That's an extra cookie.

Supplements

A ton of people take supplements—sometimes. But most of them don't make taking supplements a habit. They take them, and then they don't take them. Often they aren't even sure why they are taking what they (sometimes) take. I often see patients who are literally taking twenty to thirty different supplements. When I ask them why they're taking each one, often they say they have no idea.

Though I encourage you to use all of your other new habits

based on food and lifestyle interventions to improve your health, there are many useful supplements, too. The key here is to ask yourself, "Can I get this from food instead? What's the specific issue in my ecosystem that I want to address? And how can I measure whether or not this supplement is doing what it's intended to?" Otherwise, you could end up wasting your money.

In general, your body needs abundant B vitamins, calcium, and magnesium to have a properly functioning reproductive system. If your cycle is a total mess, start by trying to eat a few more foods high in these nutrients. What foods am I talking about? They include the following:

- **B vitamins:** Red meat, eggs, brown rice, lentils, greens, bone broth (trust me on this, it's delicious and will make your hair and nails grow like crazy), and nuts.

- **Calcium:** We all know the campaign "Milk does a body good," touting dairy products' high calcium content. The truth is that many people are sensitive to lactose and dairy products can be incredibly mucus forming, which is terrible for digestion and absorption. I recommend that folks stick to broccoli, almonds, seaweed, greens, sesame seeds (add tahini to your sandwiches), and sardines.

- **Magnesium:** Yeah, more greens and almonds. (I love to multitask.) Add in cashews, dark chocolate, and quinoa, and you'll be covered.

I don't know about you, but I would really prefer to spend my money on those delicious foods—many don't even require preparation, and they all taste great—instead of on vitamin pills.

Even in my clinic, we focus less on vitamin and mineral supplements and more on the formulas we have created to address some underlying reproductive issues. For example, if you have really serious menstrual pain, significant clotting in your menstrual blood, or really bad PMS, you might need something stronger than a vitamin in addition to lifestyle changes to correct the problem.

The formulas that we have developed are the result of more than twenty years of clinical practice by board-certified reproductive acupuncturists. Unlike minerals such as calcium and magnesium that are important for a healthy cycle, these are clinical-grade, plant-based formulas that use combinations of herbs in very high doses that are chosen to work synergistically. Plus the herbs and combinations of herbs have been proven by research to significantly improve PMS. We considered more than 17,000 studies for efficacy and safety to build the safest and most impactful formulas.

By merging our thirty years of combined clinical experience, we built a formula known for its antianxiety and antidepressant effects, as well as its ability to address the physical symptoms of PMS such as fatigue, insomnia, breast pain, anxiety, irritability, mood swings, and tension. In a study, it was proven to be effective for more than 75 percent of women, with 46.7 percent of women achieving remission of their symptoms, according to the HAM-D Depression Rating Scale . In fact, 81 percent of patients at the conclusion of the study no longer met the official criteria for PMDD listed in *Diagnostic and Statistical Manual of Mental*

Disorders, fourth edition (*DSM-IV*), the standard by which psychological issues are defined.

If you do decide to take anything in addition to lifestyle or diet changes, such as supplements, you should research them thoroughly. Not all supplements are created equal and some can be unsafe. Look for products that do more than manage symptoms, like vitex in isolation and PMS vitamin supplements, and that actually affect the root of the problem. Otherwise you could be married to those supplements until you go through menopause, and who wants that?[6]

Community Support and Connection

This last section is not likely something you think of as a habit. It's having and being engaged with a community. I call this a habit because just as with any other relationship, if you're not nurturing your relationship with your community, you're actively becoming more separated from it, and that's bad news for you, both mentally and physically. According to the Economic and Social Research Council, there are significant health costs due to social isolation. Its research found that people who have supportive friends and family generally had better mental and physical health than those who aren't as active with friends and social networks. The same was true of those who take part in churches, clubs, and voluntary organizations. As I have mentioned many times before, we live in a very individualistic culture in which it's all too easy to become focused on ourselves and our own achievements, leaving little time for friends, family, and community. But the data are clear that those relationships are essential to overall well-being.[7] We all have dreams and desires for ourselves, and that is great. What we sometimes forget is that in order to achieve something really meaningful, we need help. It's hard for women to achieve in our society in general but even harder when our community ties are weak and there are fewer people to call upon for help and support when we really need it.

Now, I know that when you don't feel good, it can be a challenge to reach out to a friend. Sometimes a date with Netflix and some boxed wine seems like the easiest choice, but although such a solution may help temporarily, in the long run, it will contribute to the continued decline of your overall health.

Remember, you are always moving in one direction or the other; you are becoming either more connected or more disconnected every day.

Becoming healthy and making changes don't have to add more stress to your life. We often think we have to do a huge overhaul to get somewhere, but all you really have to do is take a baby step. Here are a couple of ideas:

1. Schedule a twenty-minute in-person coffee date with a friend who works within walking distance of your office. Make it easy for both of you to say yes. That will give you face time with a friend as well as a little walk outside. I have had a walking date with one of my very best friends, Honey, for the last twenty years. We have changed the day a few times, but in general, whenever we're both in town, one day a week we meet downtown on the lake at 8:00

a.m. and walk the lakeside trail before we start our day. It's one of the highlights of my week, and I protect it like gold.

2. Schedule a monthly potluck at your place. Invite a few interesting people, make it BYOB, and ask folks to bring some snacks or appetizers. Even if your place is small, it's a baby step toward building a community around you.

Like the environment, we are sensitive and reactive to everything around us and inside us, to our behaviors and the behaviors of others. And, like our planet's, our individual and collective physical ecosystems are breaking down. Our diets, sleep, mind-sets, stress levels, and ability to manage our lives are all connected, and the results are expressed in our menstrual cycles.

Bottom line, our periods are like our canary in the coal mine of our world. When the canary is sick, we have to go back to good habits to create health in our personal ecosystem again. Sleep, diet, exercise—each of these seems like a separate problem to be addressed in isolation; however, they are intimately interrelated. In order to correct one, you have to look at how they're all connected and address them as a system.

For example, say you want to lose weight. You know you're consuming a diet full of things that aren't useful to your body, such as sugar, refined carbs, and booze. But you're also not sleeping enough, and when you do sleep, the quality of your rest is poor. You toss and turn all night, leaving you still tired in the morning. Guess what? It's going to be almost impossible to make sustainable behavior changes to your eating habits until you figure out what's going on with your sleep.

This perspective can be difficult to digest (pun intended!). We live in an incredibly driven culture that has consistently rewarded us for ignoring all of these holistic connections. It has trained us to take pills to solve our problems as quickly and effortlessly as possible, but that approach just doesn't work for all of us anymore. Our menstrual cycles are letting us know we are sick, and we need to start acknowledging that fact. Ignoring what our periods are telling us and pretending that we're all fine when almost no one is prevents us from thriving.

Why do we ignore our own sicknesses? Some part of ourselves knows that things aren't working. But it's like when you're in a bad relationship: you know it's bad, but doing something about it seems like too much work. We've all been there!

We get stuck because we're in conflict between our own wants and needs and the demands of society and social media. We often grapple with our desire to prove that we're worthy in a society that regularly makes us feel as though we're not good enough. We eat too little, consume low-quality food (even women who think they're eating healthier do this to themselves, drinking cold protein shakes that can be hard to digest and salads made of iceberg lettuce), or scarf down meals on the run. Our connections are with screens rather than with people. We endure significant amounts of stress in an attempt to get ahead in careers we don't really love, we're either too sedentary or exercising too much, we skimp on sleep. We're generally exhausted, but instead of sleeping, we drink too much caffeine, so much so that at bedtime we can't unwind, so we end up drinking a bunch of wine or margaritas at happy hour. (And now data show that no alcohol consumption is healthy for women.)

Of course, I'm not saying that this is every woman's lifestyle, but I *can* say that after twenty years of working with women, I've understood that some version of this is pretty close to the norm, not an outlier. That's true even for me! I struggle to focus on self-care because skimping on it often feels easier.

Healthy habits are the foundation on which our periods can flourish. And currently, the majority of periods aren't flourishing. We need both quality and quantity in our nutrients, plus the ability to digest them and convert them into energy and blood for our periods. The whole system is annihilated when we're overstressed, overexercised, or underslept. Your liver has to be able to metabolize and help eliminate your hormones, and to do its job, it relies on an adequate production of blood, which in turn depends upon digestion, and so on.

We aren't talking openly about our cycles. And when we don't talk openly, we limit access for the world to understand the impact of our suffering, which prevents us from gaining access to solutions to help us.

Take Action!

Now let's find a solution. Start tracking your habits for the next week so you can set a baseline of your behaviors.

MAPPING OUT YOUR PERSONAL PERIOD PLAN

A clear vision, backed by definite plans, gives you a
tremendous feeling of confidence and personal power.

—BRIAN TRACY

You may have noticed that I often speak about improving our menstrual cycles in terms of "fixing" them. I use this language not because menstrual cycles are "broken." But since we have been conditioned to think that everything that's going on with our cycles is peachy keen, we need to find language to talk about correcting the issues that aren't necessarily disease states but still warrant improving. It's not that you're broken, it's that you deserve to feel great every day. Like it or not, our cycles want and deserve our attention, not least of all because there's a lot that they're trying to tell us about our bodies.

Don't get me wrong; there are people suffering from many kinds of health problems whom I don't know how to help. I don't know how to help someone in intractable pain from bone cancer. I don't know how to satisfy the needs of hungry people where there is no food. I don't know how to quench people's thirst where there is no clean water. But based on my clinical experience, I'm very confident that I can reduce pain and suffering associated with menstrual disease. Throughout my life, I've always said that my purpose is to end needless suffering, and, in my opinion, menstrual pain is almost always unnecessary. The only problem is that there's not enough of me to go around! No matter how much I work, I can't fix the nearly one and a half billion menstrual cycles that are screwed up. Plus, I'd rather enable and empower *you* so that *you* have real agency over your current and future health and your fertility. That is pretty exciting work, if you ask me!

So let's dig in. In the last few years, I've met with many investors to talk about the technology that has been built to help women improve their periods and their fertility. We developed algorithms to diagnose a woman's entire health ecosystem from the data we ask her to input and then create highly customized interventions to fix her issues. Potential investors always want to know what the one or two things are that women need to do to improve their health and fertility. How can our algorithm possibly have so much impact on their overall health? They ask me, "What's the secret sauce?" And I always laugh, because they're taking such an allopathic approach, meaning that they're still looking for a one-to-one relationship, a way to "fix" a bad symptom.

So my answer is always the same: the "secret sauce" can't be boiled down into one thing. You can't just start eating more spinach to stop your cramps or quit drinking coffee and magically cure your clotting. The real power is in developing the ability to understand and assess all of the factors that are contributing to your problems and how they're related to one another. That's how you can start making the biggest difference in your health and overall ecosystem.

Finding Your Pattern

I want to give you the tools to be able to use this book as a resource to help you identify your problems and a starting point to get you going in the right direction. As you can see from what you've read so far, identifying your symptoms and how they're related, deciding how your habits are contributing to your symptoms, and figuring out the order of operations can be complicated because, well, our bodies and ecosystems are complicated. I mean that in the best way; if we weren't complicated, we would be dudes. Okay, sorry, that was a little joke. Seriously, our systems are complex because the act of making humans is sophisticated stuff. In the scope of this book, I can't teach you how to be me or mimic the algorithms I taught Brazen to perform, but I can teach you the basics by creating a few archetypes. These come straight out of Chinese medicine and can help you see some of your basic patterns and how to go about making a few changes.

Note: you are very unlikely to be just one archetype. As I said, you and your body are complex, so don't be deterred if you see some of yourself in several of the patterns. I want you to be able to understand that you're not just one symptom or another but rather groups of symptoms that are in turn parts of larger groups of symptoms. It's not unlike astronomy: there are planets that exist in the solar system, which is part of our galaxy, and so on.

I'm going to give you four archetypes to get you thinking. There are many more archetypes, and you should know that as you feel better, your pattern will change. That's a good thing. Remember when we spoke about peeling back the layers of the onion to get to the root cause of your symptoms? This is another example.

Read through the archetypes, and see which profiles seem the most like you. (You don't have to have all of the symptoms to fit into a category.) Then you can continue to read about what strategies and foods will be most supportive for your archetype(s).

Let's look at the four archetypes I see most commonly.

I'm pretty much out of gas.

You feel tired most of the time, you prefer to stay home, it takes a lot of work to motivate yourself to exercise, you have a tendency toward gas and bloating, and you have scanty and even pale menstrual blood. If you have PMS and/or cramping, it's because there simply isn't enough energy or blood to support your liver as it tries to metabolize your hormones. You may feel as though "I'm just not in good enough shape." This is super common. You think that if you work out more, you'll feel more energized, but in reality, you are just exhausted and probably running on adrenaline.

Your first steps should be:

1. **Sleep as much as humanly possible.** I'm not kidding. Anytime you can lie down and go to sleep—even if that means going to your car at lunchtime and napping there—do it. Everyone who knows me, from patients to venture capitalists, knows that if there's a will, there is a way for me to nap, and I'm going to figure it out. There is so much shame attached to resting. It looks lazy, but the reality is that the better rested you are, the better and more focused your performance will be.

2. **Eat specific foods to help you make blood.** We're talking foods with iron and vitamin B12 in them, such as organic red meat and sockeye salmon. Eggs and organic beef bone broth can also accelerate blood production. If you're vegan, this can be extremely difficult to do. Without animal products in your diet, the only source of vitamin B12 is from a supplement, which, in my clinical experience, won't cut the mustard for most women. Even vegans can, however, focus on iron-rich foods such as kale and spinach, all the dark berries, blue-green algae (take this in a tablet form—it's too gross otherwise), parsley, and the granddaddy of them all, dried apricots. Though they are too high in sugar content if you're eating keto, dried apricots have more iron per ounce than beef does.

3. **Exercise very moderately.** Your best bets will be walking, gentle yoga, and, even better, restorative yoga and

meditation. Anything more intense will just continue to empty the tank and keep you from making progress. At some point you'll start feeling stronger and may want to add a bit more exercise time and intensity. I encourage you to take your time with intensity. Just baby-step it.

I think I'm super healthy, but I'm running mostly on adrenaline and caffeine.

You probably look pretty healthy from the outside. With caffeine, you probably don't feel that tired, but you also don't sleep very well. You can get a lot of shit done, but you're often annoyed, agitated, or anxious. You have too much to do, but you try your best to cram it all in. When your period comes, there's hell to pay in the days beforehand, and your cramps could be quite intense.

Your first steps should be:

1. **Start reducing your caffeine intake.** Don't go cold turkey, because that's hard on your adrenal glands. Just start substituting a 25 percent decaf blend for the next week or two. Be gentle to your body; you don't need to hurry. Then switch to 50/50 caf/decaf, and after a few more weeks switch to 75 percent decaf. Finally, switch to straight decaf. This is essential, because until you get off caffeine, you won't be able to help your adrenal glands turn off the fire hose of adrenaline that's making you feel okay every day. Running on adrenaline can work temporarily, but over time, your cortisol level will get higher

and higher and you'll develop belly fat that is super difficult to lose. Without the caffeine to keep you pumped
up, your energy reserves will bottom out. At that point
you'll start to feel tired. This is good. It means you have
gotten to the next level, probably even crossed over into
the "Out of gas" archetype.

2. **Eat real food.** I know that seems obvious, but this
archetype often drinks a lot of smoothies and lives on
protein bars. You're moving so fast that there isn't time
for anything else. In order to start to heal your system,
your body needs a lot of vegetables and organic animal
products to make energy and blood to replenish what
has been burned out by overactivity. It doesn't have to
be fancy. Sometimes when I'm really busy, I go to the
prepared food section of my local supermarket and buy
a bunch of cooked foods to get me through the week.
Meal delivery services also make it much easier to have
healthy meals without breaking the bank or taking too
much time. If you have the time, batch cook on the weekends and freeze.

3. **Back off from your intensive exercise regime.** Your
best bets will be walking, gentle yoga, and, even better,
restorative yoga and meditation. Anything more intense
will just continue to empty the tank and keep you from
making progress. At some point, you'll start feeling
stronger and may want to add a bit more time and in-

tensity. I encourage you to take your time with intensity. Just baby-step it here.

4. **Take the right supplements.** Supplements that will really help your adrenal glands recover are astragalus, ashwagandha, and licorice. I like using a tincture because then you know that they're already properly dosed and you can just shoot a dropperful directly into your mouth.

I feel cold all the time, and I struggle with my weight.

It's the middle of summer, and you're still wearing a sweater or even a light jacket! Your feet are often cold, and you're kind of pale. You frequently feel hungry but aren't very satisfied by your food. You often have sweet cravings, and sugary food scratches the itch for a while—until the next craving. You try to lose weight, but it's very slow going. You want to work out more, but it's hard to generate the motivation. You tend to have a lot of bloating after meals and, in terms of your period, have regular bleeding but with a lot of clots and mucus. Your cycle is likely to be irregular. You have more pain than PMS but may have both.

Your first steps should be:

1. **Start focusing your diet on easy-to-digest foods and cooked foods.** Try to consume more soups (these are easy to batch cook on the weekends and freeze—you can even make just broth as a base and add ingredients such as leftover chicken and steamed vegetables dur-

ing the week). Start significantly reducing your intake of carbohydrates, including bread and sweets. Reduce your fruit consumption to one serving a day, and limit your alcohol intake. Eating more cooked foods will help you turn what you're eating into energy more effectively and allow you to extract nutrients better to produce a higher quality and quantity of blood. The more you focus on a simple low-carb/high-healthy-fat (think nuts and avocados) diet, the sooner you'll start feeling a lot more energy. Also eat more warming foods such as cinnamon, garlic, onions, and curry.

2. **Stay warm.** We talked about this before, but cold folks use up a lot of their energy just trying to stay warm. That energy is squandered when you could be using it to make more energy. Remember, it takes heat to transform food into energy, and when your body temperature is too low, food sort of percolates in your gut instead of getting the spark it needs to be powerfully metabolized.

3. **Increase your exercise.** Obviously, if you're already exercising, go back to the notes for the "Out of gas" archetype, but if not, now is the time to start walking every day. It's one of the most effective ways to begin improving your temperature and metabolism. Just take it easy. Too much is still too much. A little goes a long way. Just thirty minutes after dinner is all you need to get the benefits.

I think I'm pretty normal, but my period is still horrible every month.

This is a category that many people fall into. And it's the most dangerous one. You look really healthy on the outside. You're working out, going to yoga, drinking smoothies, and eating food, too. When you go to the doctor, he or she says, "Everything looks great."

But when I ask you about your period, you tell me that it's a catastrophe. You have an irregular cycle, your PMS is hideous, you lie down in the shower because you're bleeding and cramping so badly. But hey, that's normal, right?

Though you're a specific archetype, improving this situation is highly personal. Because this archetype's issues are often driven more by very specific diet and lifestyle habits, it's difficult to give you suggestions about where to start. You can start by taking the quiz at www.foreverbrazen.com to get some customized feedback, using the Brazen supplements formulated for PMS and cramping, working on your general lifestyle habits (as discussed in this book), or looking for a reproductive acupuncturist to help you sort out a more customized plan.

The reason this archetype is so difficult to plan for is simple: there aren't enough symptoms that group together to make it easy to create a plan of attack. That's actually a good thing. Typically, there are one or two interventions that can make a big difference in a few months, as opposed to the other archetypes, which have deeper issues to resolve.

Your Power to Change Through Mindfulness

In the previous chapter, we looked at important habits, such as sleep, nutrition, exercise, and stress management. Most of us have a sense of the areas of our lives that could use some support. We could eat better, sleep more, exercise more, and do more about managing our stress. But the idea of working to change all of these behaviors can be overwhelming to someone who's already exhausted or not feeling well. You may be afraid you simply cannot take on anything more. Or maybe you've already tried—lots of times—to change some of these behaviors and failed, so that damn little voice in your head keeps telling you you've done this before and it didn't work or it's too hard or you just can't. So you don't.

When I talk to people about the importance of their minds, they always think the mental part of improving health is a "soft science." As someone who was an acupuncturist for a long time, I'm very accustomed to working in the soft sciences. I mentioned before that when I was building my technology, investors would often ask me, "What's the one thing that makes the biggest difference in changing women's health, cycles, and infertility?" I told you that there's no real answer, but I did take the question seriously. It's a good one. So we went back and looked at the data from the clinical pilot we had done and searched for any kind of answer. We spent a lot of time and money trying to answer that question, looking at the data a million different ways. And in the end, the reality was that for the most part, nothing was more important than anything else. As I said before, there is no special sauce. Except—and this wasn't something I could necessarily say to investors, but I can say it to you—mindfulness. It tested just a little bit higher than any other intervention in making a lasting impact. You can begin to improve your habits by starting to observe your inner monologue about your health, your willpower, your ability to get shit done on your own behalf. Mindfulness is the place to start. To prove that point, I want to tell you a story.

A long time ago, I attended a workshop where the opening speaker said something to the effect of what follows, in my own words, according to my memory.

"I want to take a little time every day at the beginning of class to help everybody get into the right frame of mind. I'm going to teach you a little meditation that we'll do. But even after this class, I want you to do it every single day. It takes just five minutes. I want you to find a quiet spot every single day and light a candle. I want you to look at the flame, and as you do it, slowly breathe in and out through your nose. In and out, in and out, and as you're doing that with your eyes fixed on the flame, imagine as you breathe in that you're breathing the most insidious bone cancer in through your nose into your lungs. It's walking into your bloodstream and penetrating your marrow. But when you breathe out, I want you to imagine your bone cancer is spreading like wildfire through your marrow—let the force of your breath be the power of the bone cancer penetrating through your body. So every breath in is taking in more cancer and every breath out is spreading it even deeper." Then someone shouted from the audience, "Stop!" The speaker halted and asked the participant why he wanted to stop. The participant said, "I don't feel comfortable doing this meditation." Again the speaker asked him why. The participant said, "I'm afraid that if I do this every single day, I might actually get bone cancer." The speaker said, "Wow, that's super interesting. I wonder if anyone else feels that way, too?" He then proceeded to ask the audience members to raise their hands if they thought that if they did this meditation for five minutes every day, it could actually increase their risk of getting bone cancer—or even cause it. Amazingly, almost everyone in the room raised a hand sheepishly.

Then something interesting happened that caused me to change the way I think about the power of my mind forever. The speaker said to us, "Okay, now raise your hand if you believe that if you spent five minutes every single day looking at a candle, breathing in through your nose and out through your nose, and imagining with every breath that every single cell in your body is in absolute and perfect health, raise your hand if you believe this could transform your health." No one raised a hand. Then the speaker said, "It's so interesting that you believe that focusing your mind on something bad every single day can make something bad happen inside your body, but almost none of you believe that meditating on the power of your mind to make a positive change inside your body can do anything. I don't know about you, but the idea of doing the meditation about bone cancer honestly makes me sick to my stomach. I actually felt so powerful when I realized that while I believed my body had the ability to hurt myself, I should have confidence in my mind's ability to help my body heal, too."

My point is that you should start paying attention to your mind's reaction to the conversation we're having about health and recognize your ability to change your habits in a way that can impact it significantly.

Let's break it down into a few simple steps to give you a deeper dive and more examples.

Step 1: Identify the problems.

I know we've already talked about this, but I want to review what an ideal cycle looks like so that we can start to see how your period may be different. Please don't misinterpret this as some perfectionist goal you must attain; think of it as a state in which women can experience the most optimal health and fertility. I don't want you to be perfect. I do want you to have access to your very best health and self every single day.

The ideal menstrual cycle is twenty-eight days long. Ovulation occurs on cycle day 14, with clear and stretchy cervical discharge and no pain. There's no spotting. When you get your period, there's no PMS, no cramping, and no clotting, your blood is fresh red, and you soak a tampon or pad every four hours, no more and no less. Your energy level is at 7 or 8 out of 10. You can fall asleep and stay asleep, and you wake up feeling rested. Your mood is stable throughout the month, and you feel resilient to stress. A note about that stress: we all have stress around us every single day, and most of us probably experience too much of it, but the more robust your constitution is, the more resilient your body is. As you start to improve your cycle and your health, you'll start to notice that things that used to really stress you out will begin to have less impact.

For this step, you'll need to track information about your cycle and habits through the month. The thing to remember is that data are key. Keeping this information organized month after month will really help you start to see the patterns.

Step 2: Figure out how your symptoms are related.

In order to understand how your symptoms are related, you have to go back to the ideal cycle, your signs and symptoms, and your habits; that trio is your starting point as you begin to identify where your body is performing ideally and where there's room for improvement. Now that you have collected the data in our algorithm, you can start to see the relationships among your habits, cycles, and symptoms. You can recognize patterns in what happens before you ovulate, what happens after you ovulate, and what happens when you're bleeding.

Step 3: Identify the root causes.

Once you've categorized the good and bad according to the phases of your menstrual cycle, you can look for some of the factors that are contributing to them. Let me give you an example of what this process looks like.

A woman named Tia comes into my clinic with heavy bleeding and clotting and severe menstrual cramping. The pain is debilitating. She thinks she has endometriosis but hasn't had the laparoscopy that's needed to diagnose it. Tia's also extremely tired and irritable when she gets her period. She doesn't pay much attention to her diet because she's really busy, but she does exercise, going to spin class or CrossFit every day. She considers herself to be extremely healthy and fit. Got it? So here's how we break this down.

- Cycle parameters: Heavy bleeding, cramping, clotting, irritability

- Habits: Heavy exercise, no attention to diet

- Other signs and symptoms: Fatigue

Her chief complaint is menstrual cramping. In most situations doctors will look for a way to relieve the pain with medication or even surgery. Unfortunately, that approach fails to consider that the cramping has an underlying cause; it misses a valuable opportunity to use this symptom as a red flag that other parts of her body also need support. Though cramps are, indeed, her biggest problem (as she is experiencing debilitating and life-interrupting pain every single month), it's really important to understand that her pain is mostly a side effect—a problem that occurs because her whole system is not functioning optimally. If we can start to understand how her body is working as an ecosystem and then address that ecosystem rather than just a part of it, we can have an exponentially greater effect on her overall health.

So let's look at her whole cycle. Heavy bleeding is almost always associated with heavy clotting. Nearly every woman who has significant menorrhagia (aka heavy bleeding) will also have clots in her menstrual blood. In order to continue to work toward the root of the problem, we have to ask, Why is there such heavy bleeding?

Side note: in the next few sections of this book, you'll notice that I ask the question "Why?" over and over and over again. This is the only way to get to the root cause of any problem. Otherwise we're still just addressing the side effects of whatever the root cause is. My hope is that you will learn to ask "Why?" more often and apply this way of thinking beyond your period, extending it to many other aspects of your life.

See the next step to find out what happens to the woman in this example.

Step 4: Identify the habits that are contributing to the root cause.

Once you've identified the root cause, the next step is to look at how your habits are creating it. We generally think we create better habits as a reaction to something; for example, if we are too fatigued, we respond by resting more. In fact, it's the other way around: how you care for your body often creates the patterns of illness. If you think about it like this: "I eat junk food after ovulation because I feel so bad," you're actually positioning yourself as the victim of your own body, of your signs and symptoms. And although of course you may sometimes suffer because of your health problems, I want you to realize how much power you have to influence your own health. I know that not every person reading this book will be able to get rid of all period problems, but I hope that you will learn the tools to figure out the parts of your health that need attention and start working toward correcting them.

But back to my patient. You might be wondering how her habits contributed to the root causes of her problem. The main root cause is cold. This is very confusing for most people, because from a Western point of view, we don't talk about hot and cold being pathologies. But from a TCM perspective, when the body is too cold, it cannot generate enough heat to make energy and circulate blood, oxygen, and nutrients effectively. Sometimes this results from a constitutional problem such as hypothyroidism or even subclinical hypothyroidism (which looks like hypothyroidism but doesn't show up in lab work), habits such as eating too many cold foods (it requires heat to metabolize these, so over time, eating them a lot starts to reduce heat in the body), or drinking a lot of cold liquids (they actually lower your body temperatures). And although this might seem obvious, a biggie is not wearing enough clothing when it is cold outside. Your body needs energy to stay warm, and when it's cold out and you don't have enough warm clothes on—think no socks, low-rise jeans, no hat or scarf—your body has to use a lot of extra energy to keep you warm. Once in a while this is not a big problem, but over time your resources become depleted and you can end up taxing your whole system.

Step 5: Follow the order of operations.

All of us know that we should exercise more, eat fewer carbs and cookies, drink less wine, be less stressed, lose or gain weight, and do a host of other things we read about online. But almost none of us does it. Behavior change can be daunting, especially if there's a lot to do. Well, I've found a few secrets that can make a huge difference.

First you have to determine all of the things that are not working for you, both physical and behavioral (such as habits), and start viewing them as the *system* that you're working on improving instead of just one issue (and another issue, and another . . .). I know that at first it seems less scary to take on just one problem—such as getting more sleep—but there are a few problems with that line of thinking that can derail your efforts. If you work only on sleep and there are ten other things you also need to dig into, there's a strong chance that only your sleep patterns will change, and if you haven't changed your whole environment, you will go back to your old sleep habits in no time. But trying to take on twenty-five issues at once usually doesn't work, either. When you take on too much at once, you're likely to feel scared and overwhelmed. "How can I do all this? I'm already so busy!" This isn't because you're lazy (although it's common to feel that way when you're struggling to make behavior changes); it's actually due to the parasympathetic nervous system. As soon as you get freaked out, you go into survival mode and all you care about is not dying, so that being rational, planning for the future, staying calm, and persisting—all things essential to behavior change—go into the toilet in favor of a big dose of adrenaline. How can you prevent that from happening? By looking at the group of things that need attention—not as a big ball of stuff that you can't or don't want to do but rather as a collective opportunity. If you even make small progress on the important ones, the benefits compound across the system.

But okay, sometimes figuring out how to get started can be hard to do without a professional's guidance. So if you're doing this on your own, use this list as the order of operations and first baby steps to take. It should help you build on your successes across your body systems and see results quickly.

1. **Mind-set.** If one thing has to be first on your list, this baby is it. Mind-set is what you're telling yourself about all of your problems, and it will determine how fast you can change your habits and your health. The first step is to take a solid inventory about what you think is possible for your health (often your opinions are backed up by lots of scientific-sounding "facts" you've heard, such as "treatable only by surgery," "impossible to get pregnant," "your only option is antidepressants or birth control").

Then start paying attention to how much you look for more evidence to support that point of view and how much your words reflect being stuck where you are. It doesn't have to be a heavy blame game; you can just set a reminder on your phone a few times a day and ask yourself what you have been focusing on and what your primary emotional state was. After a week you'll start to see a very strong pattern. Then you get to choose: is that what you want to create for yourself? Or do you want to create a new focus, new thoughts, and a new emotional state? If the answer is yes to the latter, all you have to do is keep noticing the difference between your former way of being and keep comparing it to the way of thinking you want to create.

2. **Exercise.** Depending upon their level of fatigue, most women working on improving their health do best with forty-five minutes of walking five days a week and yoga three times a week. You don't have to join a gym for this; just find some good videos online and do them in your bedroom!

3. **Sleep.** Your goal is to sleep eight hours per night. Start with going to bed fifteen minutes earlier than usual and only read. I promise, if you're fatigued in general, this will help you wind down earlier.

4. **Stress.** This is a toughie, but if you've made inroads into the previous three areas, you should be ready for it. Being super stressed (which just about everyone is) will erode all of the great work you do anywhere else. It can be stressful just thinking about how stressed you are, especially if you're feeling as though you don't have the time or resources to become less stressed. Don't worry. Download the Headspace app, use it for ten minutes a day for two weeks, and see what happens. It does a brilliant job of making meditation easy—all you have to do is lie there and do what the voice says.

5. **Water.** This seems like a no-brainer, but almost every patient I have ever seen doesn't drink enough water. Easy fixes: (1) Drink one more glass of water every day. (2) Go to the sink as soon as you wake up and pound a glass or two while you wait for your coffee to brew and you will be finished drinking your water before your coffee is ready.

6. **Food quality.** Often, we focus on avoiding this or that. Certainly, sugar and alcohol (which is really just more sugar) won't do your body any good (damn), but instead of trying to restrict yourself too much in the beginning, try adding one more high-quality food to your daily diet. Choose something simple; for example, buy a bag of peeled baby carrots and take them to work. Eat one serving every day as your afternoon snack until they're gone,

even if you also have chips. Just eat the carrots first. You want to start building habits instead of trying for total transformation in one week.

Take Action!

You've identified your symptoms and your patterns; now you can take the quiz at www.foreverbrazen.com to make a plan to work on them.

8
·········

DIAGNOSIS DOESN'T MEAN YOU'RE DOOMED

'd like to talk about some of what I call "menstrual diseases." Now, that doesn't mean that all these conditions are necessarily diseases. For example, menopause is something that's going to happen to all of us if we live long enough, and it's more of a hormonal transition than a disease. However, I include it in the category of menstrual diseases because it impacts women's health and quality of life in a very significant way. Some of these conditions you should be worried about, some not, but in general, they're all things that can affect your period, your comfort, and your health in a negative way.

In each of the following sections, I'll give you a brief overview of each condition and some of the strategies you can use to improve it significantly. These strategies won't cost you anything, but you'll have to focus a little to bring them to reality. It's worth the effort, though; they can make a significant impact. If you aren't making good progress, or if you're struggling to make a behavior change on your own, I encourage you to find a qualified reproductive acupuncturist (www.aborm.org) or use the Brazen app to help.[1]

No matter what's going on with you (or not), there are some basic steps everyone can take to be healthier and feel better. Be sure to start here before you do anything else. These small changes will make the other changes easier when you get to them and will help you make faster progress in the long term. Remember, many of the diagnoses I'm going to be talking about, including infertility, are chronic conditions. Even if you're not trying to get pregnant, some underlying issues may still be running in the background of your health ecosystem. All of those issues are not only a huge pain in your—well, butt—but they also *potentially* increase your risk of developing diseases that can kill you, including heart disease, diabetes, and estrogen-dominant cancers. Even PMDD increases your risk of committing suicide, and endometriosis increases your risk of developing additional autoimmune conditions.

But don't worry, I'll give you not only research-backed information about each condition but also some high-level guidelines to help you get started. Just do me one favor: please, please, please remember that no matter how much you and everyone else wants for there to be a magic pill to solve these issues (or any of the other diseases in the world), *there just isn't one*. The magic comes from customizing a plan for exactly your situation and then working on all the aspects of your life and your body's ecosystem that contribute to your problem.

I want you to approach the issues around your health and period—whatever they are—as an opportunity.

Yes, I said opportunity. Your body is highly responsive to the world around you and to its own needs, and it's telling you the way you are caring for it is or isn't working—even if you're really trying. The body knows. Every month it's giving you tangible feedback. Even better, most of that feedback is actionable, so you can really do something about your symptoms. It sounds like a joke when I talk about the menstrual cycle and its associated challenges as women's unfair advantage. But if we never got the feedback from our bodies—and it wasn't a pretty hideous experience—we might not be inspired to do anything different, and our bodies would be getting less and less healthy every day. No one ever believes me when I say this, but as I told you, being diagnosed with MS was one of the most valuable things that ever happened in my life. Without that diagnosis, I would not have become the kind of person and clinician that I am now. I have a deep relationship with chronic illness and what it takes to transcend it. I'm deeply familiar with the feeling of hopelessness and know that it can be overcome, but it takes determination and a great road map. Without that experience, I wouldn't be writing this book—or have been able to help tens of thousands of infertile couples realize their dreams of being parents.

More important, when I go to the doctor for a checkup each year and she looks at my lab results, she is always blown away by how healthy I look on paper for a fifty-year-old—and how great I tell her I feel.

This all comes back to mind-set.

I know you may feel miserable and hopeless. Please don't let that become your habit. Remember, where the mind goes, the body follows. Each day on this journey, you have to look for what is working—even when there isn't much: try to find the wins. What you look for is what you will find. Look for progress. Look for power. Look for transcendence, even if only in baby steps. Look for it and celebrate it, and your path to recovering your health will be, as a good friend of mine says, a squillion times better.

The Starting Points

1. **Get adequate sleep.** I cannot stress enough that sleep is the best friend of anyone with almost any chronic condition. Nearly every woman I've ever worked with has been underslept. Most people think eight hours is the ideal amount, and it's certainly better than what most people are getting, but the research on sleep and athletic performance shows that people actually perform optimally at ten hours per night.[2] Almost nothing about your health can change if you're not sleeping enough. Restoration is essential to healing and positive mental health.

2. **Take any step to start managing your stress.** We talked about some strategies in the previous chapter, but if you need a baby one that's super easy, let me remind you:

just start listening to meditations on the app Headspace. It's one of the easiest tools to help you get acquainted with meditation. The key is to do it regularly. Listen at bedtime if you're having trouble falling or staying asleep. One more tip: multitasking has been shown to decrease your productivity to a level comparable to that of someone smoking pot, so do one thing at a time.

3. **Move your booty.** Yes, I know this seems obvious. What I want to reinforce here from the previous chapter is to move it just *some*: gentle, moderate movement but at least five days per week. Let me be clear: at first, more (as in "a lot of") exercise is not better. We have to break out of that mind-set. In order to heal, you *must* allow your body to rest and recover.

Now let's look at specific conditions and some precise recommendations.

Polycystic Ovarian Syndrome (PCOS)

Worldwide, about 6 percent of people with periods have PCOS, and it's a leading cause of infertility. The name can be confusing; it's generally not about cysts on your ovaries, it is more of a hormonal and metabolic condition in which your body cannot metabolize sugar effectively and starts to develop insulin resistance. In addition to affecting your blood sugar level, insulin resistance can cause an increase in your androgen (male hormone) production (think testosterone and facial hair). This condition frequently goes undiagnosed and can have an enormous effect on your well-being. Common symptoms of PCOS include irregular or missed periods due to not ovulating, fatigue, headaches, acne, excess body hair, sleep problems, and thinning head hair—all because of the increased levels of androgens and lower levels of progesterone (a female hormone). Maybe the most significant symptoms here, though, are pelvic pain and infertility.

If your doctor suspects that you have PCOS, she/he may recommend that you have a blood test to look for elevated luteinizing hormone (LH) and serum testosterone levels. She/he may also suggest an ultrasound of your ovaries to determine if cysts are present. However, about 20 percent of all women have ovarian cysts that are visible on an ultrasound; having the cysts doesn't necessarily mean you have PCOS.

If you are diagnosed with PCOS, you have some degree of estrogen dominance, which basically means too much estrogen, but as this can become so severe and impactful, it's critical to manage it first. Estrogen dominance can be the result of many different factors and is rarely related to just one thing. Remember, everything is interrelated! Estrogen dominance may be caused by any one or a combination of the following: your ability to metabolize hormones is sluggish; your progesterone level is low; you've taken hormonal birth control; you've been exposed to a lot of xenoestrogens (compounds that mimic estrogen), such as those found in fragrances, solvents, plastics, parabens, and pesticides; or you are approaching menopause. When you combine those factors, the risk goes up.

There are lots of people out there who don't have clinical PCOS, but their presentation looks a heck of a lot like that of PCOS. They may have some of the symptoms, such as unwanted facial hair, difficulty losing weight, and irregular periods or ovulation. Those people are probably on their way to PCOS but have a great opportunity to stop the progress. Following the suggestions below, as everyone who does have PCOS should, will be incredibly beneficial to them, too.

Diagnosis or not, individuals with PCOS or (in my opinion) look-alike patterns should be aware that this metabolic syndrome increases your risk of developing some pretty serious conditions, such as heart disease, depression, diabetes, stroke, and estrogen-dominant tumors such as breast and ovarian cancers. You will also have an increased risk for weight gain and difficulty losing weight, hyperinsulinemia, hyperlipidemia, and eating disorders.

Self-Care Specifics for PCOS

- **Manage your weight.** This is easy to say and hard to do for many people but especially for a woman with PCOS because her hormones are working against her. Losing just 10 percent of your body weight can have a large enough impact on your hormone levels to modulate your ovulation cycles and help get your period back on track. I know that being told to lose weight can feel like a double whammy because it's so hard to do, but fat is a big part of what's contributing to the hormone imbalance, because estrogen and androgens are stored in fat.

So even though it's tough, by reducing your overall fat stores, you can significantly reduce the number of hormones circulating in your body.

- **Move for thirty minutes every day.** This is a little more vigorous than what I recommend for everyone else but still not crazy hard. Research shows that thirty minutes of daily brisk walking, swimming, or yoga can help manage the symptoms of diabetes and improve insulin sensitivity, as well as help with weight control.

- **Eat to improve your hormone metabolism and elimination.** The hormones in the foods you might be eating are the first place to start. Make sure that the animal products you are consuming are organic and hormone free. This is especially true of high-fat animal products such as butter and cheese. Remember that hormones are stored in fat. If you're consuming high-fat foods from an animal that has been inoculated with a ton of growth hormone, you're exposing yourself and your already taxed hormone system to a large and unnecessary burden.

- **Eat the following cruciferous vegetables** to help you metabolize excess estrogen in the body.

  - Broccoli
  - Cauliflower

- Kale

- Watercress

- Brussels sprouts

- Cabbage

- **Eat the following fibrous foods,** which will encourage your body to excrete excess hormones and help slow the absorption of glucose in the intestines.

  - Lentils, white beans, black beans, kidney beans, garbanzo beans, edamame

  - Whole grain oats and oatmeal

  - Artichokes

  - Peas

- **Regulate your blood sugar and glucose metabolism.** This is pretty much a *must* for all PCOS patients, overweight or not, and one that they all need to address to prevent insulin resistance and impaired glucose metabolism. You should avoid simple and refined sugars and focus your carb intake on unrefined complex carbohydrates with a low glycemic index. Combine these carbohydrates with proteins or fats for optimal breakdown and metabolism.

I know this all sounds complicated, but it really isn't. For the most part you want to seriously look at cutting out refined sugar and carbohydrates altogether. This includes keeping your fruit consumption to one small serving a day. Though fructose is a natural sugar, it will still spike your blood sugar level. All sugars and refined carbs will work against you and your efforts to get your blood sugar and health under control. So making this change is the single most important way to prevent your PCOS from turning into diabetes.

Here are a few examples. Sadly, these foods include so many things that many of us really enjoy eating, including most white foods like pasta, bread, and rice, as well as my beloved cake, processed cereal, and soda. I see a lot of people substituting diet drinks for sugary soda, and I want to caution against this. In my opinion, artificial sweeteners in diet drinks are probably worse for you than sugar. Studies show that people who drink diet drinks are on average 10 pounds heavier than those who do not.[3] You might be thinking "Well, maybe that's because they're already overweight and are drinking diet sodas to help lose weight," but the research shows that artificial sweeteners may also actually trigger elevations of blood sugar level.[4] Researchers have found that the consumption of saccharin, sucralose, and aspartame raises blood sugar level by dramatically changing the makeup of the gut microorganisms, mainly bacteria, that are in the intestines and help with digestion and the immune system.[5] Other research has suggested a link between diet soda consumption and an elevated risk of stroke.[6]

Keep your diet healthy and balanced. Here are some useful suggestions.

- Eat at least five servings a day of vegetables, including two of leafy greens.

- Eat one-half cup of legumes, such as black beans or lentils, daily.

- Enjoy grass- or pasture-fed meat up to three times a week.

- Choose berries as your fruit when you can—they have a lower glycemic impact than other fruit.

- Pay careful attention to portion sizes in order to moderate your glucose load and minimize insulin resistance.

- Add cinnamon to your coffee to help decrease your insulin resistance.

- Consume prebiotic and probiotic foods, which promote the growth of beneficial bacteria in the intestinal tract. Prebiotics are found in whole grains, onions, bananas, garlic, honey, leeks, artichokes, and some fortified foods. Probiotic foods include fermented foods (sauerkraut, live-culture yogurt, kimchi, miso).

- Eat lots of healthy fats, such as avocados; nuts and seeds and their butters; olive, sesame seed, and coconut oil; and cold-water fish: anchovies, sardines, mackerel, trout, sockeye salmon.

- Take a few supplements to help manage your blood sugar. These include:

  - Chlorophyll, which reduces symptoms of hypo-glycemia (low blood sugar) without raising blood glucose level.

  - B vitamins, magnesium, alpha-lipoic acid, and conjugated linoleic acid improve insulin resistance.[7]

  - N-acetylcysteine (NAC), which regulates blood sugar and is a strong antioxidant.

  - Saw palmetto, which blocks the production of dihydrotestosterone (DHT).

  - Bitter melon and fenugreek, which regulate blood glucose level.

  - 2 × 2,000 milligrams myoinositol plus 2 × 200 micrograms folic acid per day, which is a safe and promising tool for the effective improvement of symptoms and infertility for patients with PCOS.[8]

The Keto Diet and PCOS

You may have heard of people talking about the keto diet as a way to lose weight quickly while still eating lots of butter and cheese. Well, both of those things are true, but there is much more to this way of eating, and it is making a huge impact on people with diabetes in terms of insulin management. I recommend most of my patients with PCOS consider doing the ketogenic diet for ninety days (after consultation with their doctor) and monitor what happens to their cycle, and PCOS symptoms. Following a keto diet is a way of training your body away from using glucose (sugar, which it's been using your whole life) as a fuel and helping it transition to using fat as its fuel source instead. There are many books and resources that can teach you about the keto diet, and if you're considering using it to manage your weight and blood sugar, I encourage you to visit this website: www.ruled.me. It's a great primer and tool kit to get you started.

Most people with PCOS who have tried the keto diet have had life-changing experiences around their health and cycles. For the first time, their bodies have a fuel source that they can use, they can lose weight, and typically they feel great.

However, here are a few notes to keep in mind about the keto diet. The first few weeks can be rough as your body is transitioning from using sugar to using fat as energy. You can feel kind of sick for as long as two weeks. Stay the course. Once your body switches over, you'll feel great. There are a bunch of myths about keto—such as "Just eat meat and fat, and everything will be fine." Not true. You need to figure out what macronutrients you need. Ruled.me has a great calculator, and you need to eat according to what the calculators say to ensure that you get enough fat and protein and the right number of calories.

Endometriosis

This common hormonal and immune condition affects an estimated one in ten women. It's named after the endometrial tissue, which lines the uterus and is discarded in your monthly period, and then grows again. In endometriosis, some of this tissue grows outside your uterus—sometimes on the ovaries, fallopian tubes, or the outside of your uterus. Because this tissue, like your uterine lining, responds to your changing hormones, it may also shed and bleed when you have your periods. The "nodules," as they're sometimes called, can cause (often intense) pain and infertility. They also create an elevated risk of developing a variety of other diseases, including some immune diseases such as multiple sclerosis and rheumatoid arthritis, as well as heart disease, so there's a lot of incentive to get to the root of the problem and address it.

Endometriosis pain has been compared to the pain of a heart

attack—and that's something you should act on. It's a progressive disease that will get worse the longer you ignore it. You may not need surgery, but you should certainly take the condition seriously and work in concert with your doctor to make sure you're taking the best steps toward better health.

Here are a few other things you should know about endometriosis that not many people are talking about. Endometriosis has a genetic link and is six times as likely to occur in women who have a mother or sister with the disease. That may support the theory that endometriosis may have an autoimmune component.

Endometriosis is also more common in women who have never given birth or who become pregnant for the first time later in life. We know that many conditions related to reproduction significantly improve after the birth of a child. I often hear physicians telling women with endometriosis, "Just have a baby, and then everything will be fine." I think it's just about the worst advice you could possibly give someone! Bringing a child into the world is a huge undertaking, and using it as a way to treat disease is probably the wrong reason to do it. Plus many women have gotten pregnant and *not* seen any improvement in their endometriosis.

So if having a baby or, for that matter, having surgery isn't an option you want to choose to manage your endometriosis, here are some others. These personal care ideas are in no way meant to be cures for endometriosis, but they can significantly improve the presentation and symptom management of the disease.

Self-Care Specifics for Endometriosis

- Like PCOS, endometriosis can be sensitive to estrogen dominance, so eat a low-carb, high-healthy-fat diet with plenty of fiber. This can make a significant impact, due to the inflammatory nature of the disease.

- Increase your intake of liver-friendly foods such as kale, Brussels sprouts, and broccoli.

- Avoid gluten. Studies have shown significant reductions in pain in some individuals with endometriosis when they stuck to a gluten-free diet for twelve months. I also recommend that you get tested for other food sensitivities. There are home tests offered by companies like EverlyWell (www.everlywell.com).

- Use anti-inflammatory spices such as turmeric (which protects against environmental carcinogens), ginger, milk thistle seeds, dandelion leaves, and ground flaxseed.

- Avoid sugar, caffeine, and alcohol.

- Avoid or minimize your consumption of dairy products since they can contribute to inflammation.

- Take N-acetylcysteine (NAC). In a 2013 study of 92 Italian women with endometriomas who took 600 milligrams of NAC three times per day for three days each week, 24 experienced a decrease in their pain levels and shrinkage of the endometriomas. Fifty-five percent of those patients reported a decrease in dysmenorrhea, or painful periods, 50 percent reported a decrease in menstrual pain, and 59 percent a decrease in chronic pelvic pain.[9]

- Though I'd prefer you to get most of your nutrients from food, supplementing with vitamins B, C, and E can help your body with oxidative stress and hormone metabolism, which should aid in decreasing endometriosis pain.

- Get acupuncture. Studies have shown that it can improve blood flow, reduce inflammation, and decrease pain.[10]

- Use Chinese herbs. Studies have shown Chinese herbs to be more effective than some drug therapies in relieving pain and shrinking the endometrial masses.[11] You can start with Brazen Cramp Support, and if you need additional support, you can contact a board-certified reproductive acupuncturist at www.ABORM.org.

- Use hot castor oil packs on your lower abdomen. These can bring relief from endometriosis pain if used regularly. There are very little data proving that doing so is impactful, but the majority of patients I have worked with get tremendous relief by soaking a small towel in castor oil, placing a heating pad on top (protected by a plastic bag), and resting with their legs up for an hour.

ORAL CONTRACEPTIVES AND ENDOMETRIOSIS

As discussed earlier in this book, taking birth control pills is a very common approach to managing painful period symptoms. But as I also said before, this will at best only manage the symptoms and can actually mask the signals your body is sending you that something is really wrong. I would venture to say that probably thousands of women come to my clinic having tried to get pregnant after being on the pill for a long time only to find that when they went off it, their symptoms had gotten much worse—and suddenly they couldn't get pregnant, either.

So although your doctor may suggest taking the birth control pill continuously for several months to stop your periods altogether, and though I know that can be a tremendously welcome break in the cycle of pain for many women, please consider it very carefully. The problem with this mode of treatment is that it doesn't solve the underlying cause of your pain, the endometriosis! It only stops you from getting your period. As soon as you quit taking the birth control pill and your periods return, the pain and other symptoms can also return. It is important to discuss the pros and cons with your doctor.

Premenstrual Dysphoric Disorder (PMDD)

PMDD is a mood disorder that's sparked cyclically by the hormones you produce before your period and usually subsides once you start bleeding. An estimated 5 to 10 percent of women of reproductive age experience this reaction. To be clear, this isn't the result of a hormone imbalance—it's a response to the hormones your body "normally" produces.

PMDD causes intense symptoms in the luteal phase (just before your period). You may feel sad, depressed, tense, anxious, irritable, or angry. You may find that you're more likely to cry, you may have more trouble focusing or sleeping, and you may feel less interested in your daily life. Physically, you may get bloated, your breasts may feel tender, or you may have headaches or achy muscles. And you may just feel exhausted.

But it's worse than plain old PMS. Think of PMDD as PMS on crack. The worst kind of crack. The kind that makes women feel so awful that 15 percent of them will attempt to kill themselves. Many are misdiagnosed with bipolar disorder as well because of the cyclical nature of their condition.

We don't know the exact mechanism behind PMDD, but it's generally accepted that hormone changes can cause a drop in serotonin level, which in turn causes mood to shift. New research is showing a possible connection between our genotypes and our estrogen receptors.[12] This may also show that PMDD has a genetic component. But regardless of what's behind it, for now, let's concentrate on doing what we can to help the symptoms.

Self-Care Specifics for PMDD

- **Make sure you poop every day.** This is important for everyone working on having better periods, but if you have PMDD, it can have a significant impact. Eliminating excess hormones through your intestinal tract can improve your body's ability to metabolize estrogen. Fiber is essential for this. Some things you can do are:

  - Eat extra veggies.

  - Drink more water.

  - Take a tablespoon of apple cider vinegar before meals.

  - Consume plenty of fermented foods to support healthy intestinal flora.

- **Take supplements.** Generally it's better to get nutrients from your food, but sometimes you need the extra strength and purity you can get in a pill.

  - Taking up to 100 milligrams of vitamin B6 per day helps reduce PMS and PMDD symptoms.[13]

  - Supplementing with 2 milligrams of thiamine (vitamin B1) and 2.5 milligrams of riboflavin (vitamin B2) reduces the risk of PMS.

- Taking magnesium supplements reduces PMS/PMDD symptoms, improving mood swings. Researchers have found that women who experienced PMS had a lower magnesium concentration in their red blood cells than women who did not. I suggest using a topical magnesium spray at night before bed. This seems to be the easiest for most people to absorb.[14]

- Supplementing with calcium D-glucarate (CDG), as excess estrogen is a significant contributor to PMS/PMDD, can help support the detoxification of your liver. Take 1,000 milligrams divided into two doses on cycle days 10 to 16, when your estrogen levels are highest.[15]

- Supplementing with 1,200 milligrams of krill oil per day (it's more sustainable and cheaper and works better than omega-3 fish oil) will help treat PMS/PMDD symptoms. Consider the following symptoms:[16]

  - Depression
  - Nervousness
  - Anxiety
  - Lack of focus
  - Bloating

- Headache
- Tender breasts

All these symptoms? Looks pretty much like the list of symptoms for PMS/PMDD, right? Almost all of them have been shown to improve when you add omega-3 fatty acids or krill oil to your diet. It won't work immediately, but stick with it. The research indicates that the longer you take it, the greater the impact.

- **Be mindful.** I know I've said it before, but it bears repeating because it's important, especially for those with PMS or PMDD. Research shows that mindfulness practice significantly impacts PMS symptoms.[17,18]

Infertility

You might be thinking "Hmmm, I thought we were talking about menstrual diseases." But your fertility is the end product of how well all of your reproductive systems are functioning. Any of the conditions we are discussing here will impact your ability to become and stay pregnant.

First, what does it actually mean to be infertile? Infertility is defined as the inability to conceive after one year of unprotected intercourse (after six months if the woman is over thirty-five) or the inability to carry a viable pregnancy to live birth.[19] As of 2010, the last year for which data is available, the Centers for Disease Control and Prevention estimated that about 6.7 million

American women suffered from infertility. About 12 percent of US males ages twenty-five to forty-four (roughly 4 million men) experience some form of infertility, too.[20]

Well-known infertility treatments such as in vitro fertilization (IVF) and intrauterine insemination (IUI) can be frighteningly expensive. IVF costs an average of $22,000 per cycle, and generally two or more cycles are necessary to achieve pregnancy. The cost of medications may be as much as $5,000 to $8,000 more per cycle. That may explain why assisted reproductive technologies such as IVF are used in less than 3 percent of infertility cases. And despite their high emotional and financial costs and invasive and time-intensive treatment regimens, the current success rates of IVF in the United States remain low (about 30 percent across all cycles in 2012—see table below), but especially for women over thirty-five years of age.[21]

IVF Live-Birth Rates per Cycle by Age, 2012[22]

Age	Percentage of Cycles Resulting in Live Births
<35	40.7
35–37	31.3
38–40	22.2
41–42	11.8
>42	3.9

Add to that the fact that only about 25 percent of US insurance plans cover infertility services. Coverage for these services is not mandated by the majority of US states or by the Affordable

Care Act, often putting the financial burden of treatments solely on the shoulders of couples trying to get pregnant.

Sounds grim, right? You have to remember, too, that your fertility changes over your lifetime. Fertility is a continuum, and many factors may influence it at any given point. Some of those factors (blocked fallopian tubes, for instance) are out of your control, but many are within your control. By understanding where you fall on the fertility continuum and why you're there, you can take action to increase your chances of conception.

First things first, though. If you are struggling to conceive, it is important to have a fertility workup with a fertility doctor. You will want to have cycle day 3 labs that include FSH, Estradiol (E2), and AMH to determine the state of your hormones and how your ovaries are aging; a Hysterosalpingogram (HSG) test, which checks to see that your fallopian tubes are open; and if you have a male partner, he should have a semen analysis to make sure he has adequate numbers and quality of sperm. This will rule out any conditions that no amount of wellness, diet, or lifestyle will correct.

We need to focus on three main areas:

- Menstrual cycle characteristics

- Modifiable lifestyle factors

- Mindfulness and stress management

Maintaining an ideal cycle has never been more important than in improving your natural ability to conceive, so we are going to review it a little more in-depth and look at how it relates to your fertility with the data to back it up.

Menstrual cycle characteristics, including cycle regularity, cycle length, the amount and quality of menstrual blood, and other symptoms such as PMS and cramping are significantly indicative of your fertile potential and odds of conceiving on a cycle-to-cycle basis. What does peer-reviewed medical research say about the optimal cycle? It should be:

- **Regular.** Regular cycles increase your likelihood of conception and make timing ovulation and intercourse more reliable. On average, women with irregular cycles had only a 25 percent chance of getting pregnant each month as compared with those with more normal cycles.[23]

- **About twenty-eight days long.** A cycle of optimal length allows plenty of time for the egg to mature properly and supports a healthy window for implantation. Both shorter and longer cycles have been associated with reduced fertility, in some cases decreasing the chance of pregnancy by up to 50 percent.[24]

  As I touched on earlier, short cycles are especially detrimental to conception. In a series of studies from 1992 to 2003, researchers found that early ovulation resulted in a significant reduction (50–75%) in clinical and viable pregnancy rates.[25, 26] However, when ovulation was regulated, pregnancy rates returned to normal levels.

- **With a four-day period.** The length of your period is a good indicator of the health of your uterine lining, which enables the implantation and nourishment of a fertilized embryo. Insufficient bleeding or bleeding that lasts too long are both associated with a decreased chance to conceive, in some cases cutting your chance to conceive by half.[27]

- **With sufficient bleeding.** It's normal to soak a pad or tampon about every four hours during your heaviest menstrual bleeding. Healthy menstrual bleeding is the reflection of a healthy uterine lining. Menstrual bleeding that is scanty or too heavy indicates a lower chance of conception.[28]

- **Free of uncomfortable symptoms.** PMS, pain, cramping, and clotting are more than just uncomfortable symptoms around your period; they may indicate larger problems such as polyps, fibroids, endometriosis, or hormonal imbalances. In addition to being a drag, infertile women report these types of symptoms in much higher numbers than their fertile counterparts.[29]

Self-Care Specifics for Infertility

Lifestyle matters when it comes to getting pregnant. When you're struggling to get pregnant, continuing to try methods that have previously been unsuccessful can be a frustrating exercise in futility. By changing your behaviors, you will give yourself a better chance at changing your outcome.

- **Lifestyle.** A growing body of medical literature suggests that what you eat and drink, your weight, how much you exercise, your daily stress levels, your use of caffeine, tobacco, and alcohol, and your personal environment can all affect not only your ability to conceive but the health of any future children.

- **Diet.** A whole-food, plant-based diet has been demonstrated time and again to have not only a beneficial effect on overall health but a direct effect on a woman's fertility—particularly on regulating ovulation.[30]

    - **Why plant-based?** In a large-scale study of women who had difficulty conceiving, Harvard scientists found that increasing the intake of animal protein, even by as little as one serving a day, resulted in a 32 percent higher likelihood of ovulatory infertility. Furthermore, researchers found that women who consumed plant proteins (instead of animal proteins) for as little as 5 percent of their total daily calories had a 50 percent decrease in their risk of ovulatory infertility.[31, 32, 33, 34]

- **Whole foods, whole fertility.** A low glycemic load, such as that created by low-carbohydrate and whole-grain diets, appears to protect fertility. Women with a high glycemic load, the result of a diet high in processed and refined foods, have been demonstrated in at least one study to have nearly twice the risk of ovulatory infertility.[35]

- **Healthy fats.** In one recent study, every 2 percent increase in calories consumed via unhealthy trans fats increased the risk of ovulatory infertility by more than 70 percent. This was especially true when trans fats replaced fertility-friendly mono-unsaturated fats. That means that as little as one teaspoon of unhealthy fat can significantly impact your fertility.[36]

- **Hydration.** Every day we need to take in enough fluids to replace what is lost through breathing, sweat, and urination. We can find these fluids in the foods we eat and the beverages we drink. Not drinking enough water—or drinking too many unhealthy beverages such as soda, coffee, or alcohol—can lead to dehydration and have negative effects on your fertility.[37]

- **Effects of dehydration.** This can affect both the body and the mind. Even mild levels of dehydration have been shown to negatively affect cognitive problem solving, mood, and attentiveness and increase sensitivity to pain, as well as cause constipation, headaches, and muscle cramps.[38]

- **Healthier cervical fluid.** The more hydrated your cervical mucus is, the easier it is for sperm to get through it. Although a variety of factors determine cervical fluid viscosity, research shows that sperm have the greatest difficulty traveling through thick cervical mucus with a low water content. In other words, your staying hydrated can improve sperm's ability to fertilize your egg.[39]

- **Coffee.** Women who consume more than 100 milligrams of caffeine a day—the equivalent of 1 cup of premium coffee—were more likely to experience difficulty conceiving and higher rates of miscarriage during pregnancy.[40, 41, 42]

- **Sodas and soft drinks.** According to the Harvard Nurses' Health Study, women who consumed two or more sodas a day were up to 50 percent more likely to experience ovulatory infertility than were women who drank less than one soda a week. [43]

- **Alcoholic beverages.** Consumption of alcohol can have various effects on fertility, including increased time to become pregnant, decreased probability of conception (by more than 50 percent), abnormal blastocyst (embryo) development, and decreased embryo implantation rate, thus increasing the risk of both miscarriage and fetal death. [44, 45, 46]

- **Sleep.** If your sleep is interrupted or insufficient, your hormone function is disturbed, affecting both your fertility and your ability to function the next day.

  - **Sleep, stress, and fertility.** People experiencing either acute or prolonged sleep deprivation experience higher levels of stress and elevated levels of the associated stress hormones, such as cortisol, the following day. Elevated cortisol level relates to negative feelings of stress throughout the day and can reduce the chances of successful embryo implantation. Elevated cortisol level has also been associated with higher levels of early pregnancy loss. According to a 2009 study published by the National Academy of Sciences, pregnancies exposed to higher levels of cortisol were 2.7 times as likely to end in miscarriage.[47]

- **Sleep and hormone regulation.** Sleeping less than seven to eight hours per night has been associated with depressed leptin levels throughout the following day. Leptin is important because it influences important hormones for regulating the menstrual cycle. Furthermore, disturbances in leptin concentrations have been linked with poor egg quality.[48, 49, 50]

- **A healthy, fertile weight.** Excess body weight can have significant effects on health, increasing the risk of developing cardiovascular disease, diabetes, and even infertility/subfertility.

  - It takes longer for obese women to become pregnant. Additionally, they experience higher rates of recurrent and early miscarriages than women of normal body weight.[51, 52]

  - A lower ongoing pregnancy rate—the carrying of a fetus to term—of 38.3 percent per cycle has been found in overweight women compared to 45.5 percent per cycle in non-overweight women.[53]

- The negative effects of obesity on female fertility have been shown to be reversible. A.M. Clark and his associates found that after losing an average of 10.2 kilograms (22.5 pounds) of body weight, 90 percent of previously anovulatory obese women began ovulating again. In other words, when obese women lost weight, their cycles began to return to normal.[54]

- **Exercise.** Anywhere from one to five hours of moderate exercise per week has been significantly associated with an 18 percent average increase in women's ability to become pregnant regardless of their initial weight, though overweight and obese women showed more benefits.[55] However, overexercising has been linked to infertility. Lean women who exercised at high intensity five or more days a week have been shown to be 2.3 times as likely to develop fertility difficulties as those who did not.[56]

- **Traditional Chinese Medicine (TCM).** This has been used for thousands of years to regulate menstruation and improve fertility. New research is beginning to quantify the effect of TCM supplements on both female and male fertility.[57, 58]

  A 2015 study at the National Institute of Integrative Medicine of Australia described a meta-analysis of 40 randomized control trials involving more than 4,247 women with infertility. The review suggested that management of female infertility with Chinese herbal medicine can improve pregnancy rates twofold within a three-to-six-month period compared with Western medical fertility drug therapy. In addition, fertility indicators such as ovulation rates, cervical mucus score, biphasic basal body temperature, and appropriate thickness of the endometrial lining were positively influenced by TCM therapy, indicating an ameliorating physiological effect conducive to a viable pregnancy.

Another review (in 2013) found that using TCM in combination with IVF resulted in significant increases in the clinical pregnancy rate and ongoing pregnancy rates. However, the authors found that many studies had a high risk of bias and recommended further research.

As mentioned earlier, the third area to emphasize when trying to improve fertility is mindfulness, or what I like to call a conceivable mind.

Women with an infertility diagnosis often have higher levels of stress, anxiety, and depressive symptoms than do fertile women.[59] These symptoms are not to be taken lightly; women experiencing these symptoms can benefit from counseling or therapy.

Multiple studies have shown how unregulated stress and anxiety may be detrimental to fertility. For instance:

- The presence of stress has been demonstrated to significantly reduce the probability of conception during every day of the fertile window.[60]

- The fertilization rate of eggs decreases as the woman's stress levels increase.[61]

- Higher levels of mental stress are associated with a longer time to pregnancy, increasing the risk of infertility.[62]

- Though high levels of stress and anxiety have been correlated with an increased chance of stillbirth, maintaining a positive mood and outlook has been correlated with increased chances of delivering a live baby.[63]

Research has illustrated a fundamental link between thought patterns and the experience of stress levels. Understanding the mechanisms governing this mind/body association may have important implications for understanding and counteracting the high incidence of stress-related disorders.[64] Evidence indicates that positive mind/body activities have been found to yield improvements in cortisol levels, which can have an inverse impact on progesterone levels, making both getting and staying pregnant difficult.[65]

Increasing mindfulness and acceptance skills, as well as cognitive detachment from thoughts and feelings, helps women process negative inner states in new ways, decreasing their entanglement with them and thus their psychological distress. Data suggest that a mindfulness-based program is an effective psychological intervention for women experiencing infertility.[66]

Menopause

First of all, menopause is not a disease. It is a significant hormonal transition. Sadly, so many women suffer through this transition. Every woman, if she lives long enough, will go through menopause, a period during which she stops being reproductive and her period ceases (once you haven't had a period for a year, you're officially considered menopausal). Why am I talking to you about your period and menopause? The process can take up to several years, and during that time, your body goes through a lot of changes and your period may as well. Most women reach menopause between the ages of 45 and 55 (the average age is 51), and although some have few symptoms, others may have hot flashes, short-term memory issues, sleeping problems, and vaginal dryness. It is also important to know that perimenopause can begin around thirty-five. This is a time in which your cycle starts to change. Your flow can either increase or decrease significantly, your cramping can increase, and most often, women will start experiencing more PMS and even a resurgence of acne (really?).

Again, though each person will benefit from a customized program, this guideline is a great start. A systems approach has been validated numerous times in comprehensive clinical trials showing that good lifestyle habits, including regular exercise, sleep management, optimal nutrition, healthy relationships, social support, and relaxation, can be effective for the treatment of menopausal symptoms and other effects of aging.

Here are some things to avoid.

- **Packaged foods.** I cannot stress this enough. There is so much crap in processed foods that will make you suffer needlessly. They contain added sugar, chemical preservatives, high amounts of sodium, and synthetic additives. Typically high in carbs, which exacerbate hormone imbalances, they may also contain GMO ingredients.

- **Added sugar.** I love it. You love it. But your reproductive body, especially your perimenopausal-to-menopausal body, doesn't. It can cause weight gain (which is already a struggle), digestive issues, worsened hormone imbalances, and yeast overgrowth, causing an increase in your hot flashes and other symptoms.

- **Sweetened carbonated drinks (not just carbonated water).** Basically sugar in a can but worse. Carbonated soda and other sugary drinks deplete the body of calcium and contribute to osteoporosis, bone loss, and teeth problems. Your bones are critically important now. One in three women in nursing homes is there due to a hip fracture. Yikes! Protect those bones as if they were gold.

- **Conventional meat.** Conventional (farm-raised) meat or poultry contains added hormones that can cause problems, including increased inflammation. Remember our conversation about hormones being stored in fat. You want more hormones, but not synthetic ones that will make your symptoms worse and hurt your overall health. Instead, choose hormone-free, grass-fed, cage-free, or pasture-raised animal proteins whenever possible. Buying organic meat, eggs, dairy products, and poultry is another layer of protection that ensures that you won't be consuming antibiotics, GMO-fed meat, and added hormones.

- **Refined oils and fried foods.** Sunflower, corn, safflower, soybean, and canola oil are all high in omega-6 fats (not to be confused with omega-3s), which can contribute to inflammation and other health problems. Fried foods and trans fats are also tied to heart problems, weight gain, diabetes, and cognitive impairments, all of which are areas we need to pay attention to as we age.

- **Alcohol.** Drinking more than a moderate amount of alcohol can aggravate hot flashes and contribute to weight gain.

Some supplements have been shown to help menopausal symptoms.[67] Of course, let your doctor know if you want to start taking any of these to make sure they won't interact with your medications. Here is a list.

- **Black cohosh** (80 milligrams once or twice daily). This can help prevent menopausal symptoms, including hot flashes and night sweats. Research shows that it might also help improve sleep quality, reduce hormonal imbalances tied to diabetes or fibroids, and even help women with fertility prior to menopause.[68]

- **Vitex or chasteberry** (160 to 240 milligrams daily). Vitex has been clinically proven to relieve hot flashes. It also has many of the same hormone-balancing properties as black cohosh, helping to regulate hormones tied to sleep problems, fibroids, skin changes, and irregular periods. Research shows that vitex increases luteinizing hormone level, modulates prolactin level, and aids in the inhibition of the release of FSH, all of which help balance the ratio of progesterone to estrogen, even slightly raising the level of progesterone.[69, 70] While I don't recommend using vitex for regulating your period, I do find it useful for women to use for the transition period of menopause. In this situation, it is used as symptom relief for hot flashes, not as a solution to address an underlying condition. It is important to remember that the majority of symptoms women experience during menopause are associated with their bodies attempting to adjust to the new levels of hormones, not because there are underlying issues (like digestive issues or hormonal/liver functions) that need to be addressed in order to provide relief.

- **American ginseng** (600 to 1,200 milligrams daily). For thousands of years, ginseng has been used to increase energy and sexual arousal. Some research suggests that it can help relieve hot flashes, fatigue, depression, cognitive impairments, and vaginal dryness.[71]

- **Red clover.** This can help prevent loss of bone density and lower the risk of heart complications. Red clover contains isoflavones that can reduce symptoms related to estrogen loss, such as hot flashes, trouble sleeping, weight gain, bone loss, bone fractures or osteoporosis, cardiovascular problems, and inflammation of the joints.[72]

- **St-John's-wort.** This herb has been safely used for more than two thousand years, often to decrease anxiety, depression, and sleep-related problems. It may help stabilize your mood, reduce inflammation, improve your sleep, and make the emotional/mental transition through menopause a bit easier.[73]

- **Maca root** (1,000 to 2,000 milligrams daily). As an adaptogen herb, maca has been used for thousands of years to lower the effects of stress and aging on the body by decreasing cortisol levels.[74] It can help reduce hot flashes, low energy/fatigue, restlessness, and weight gain while improving libido and energy. I have found the brand Femmenessence MacaPause to be the most effective.

- **Adaptogen herbs.** Ashwagandha, medicinal mushrooms (not *those* kinds of shrooms), rhodiola, and holy basil can help improve thyroid function, lower cholesterol levels, reduce anxiety and depression, reduce brain cell degeneration, and stabilize blood sugar and insulin levels.

- **Brazen PMS Support.** This is a proven clinical-grade, plant-based herbal supplement formula known for its antianxiety and antidepressant effects, as well as its ability to address the physical symptoms of PMS such as fatigue, insomnia, breast pain, anxiety, irritability, mood swings, and tension.

- **Essential fatty acids.** Borage oil or evening primrose oil can help moisten tissues and prevent vaginal dryness as well as balance hormones.[75, 76]

- **Zinc.** This increases progesterone level and decreases estrogen level. In addition, it can help boost the immune system. Zinc also helps build strong bones, thereby reducing the risk of osteoporosis.[77]

- **Vitamin E.** This fat-soluble vitamin can help balance volatile hormones.[78]

- **Flaxseed oil.** This has been shown to reduce cholesterol and mood swings by improving hormonal regulation.

- **Calcium.** This should be taken starting in perimenopause to prevent postmenopausal osteoporosis.

I know that I've given you a lot to think about—and do and eat. I don't want it to seem overwhelming. But as you get started, I think you'll find that everything you do will begin to make you feel better. And the better you feel, the easier it will be to make more changes that support your health—until the improvements become exponential. And then, well, then we'll get back to taking over the world.

Take Action!

Actually, I think there's already enough for you to do in this chapter!

9

....

BEFORE I GO, A FEW VERY IMPORTANT THINGS EVERY WOMAN SHOULD KNOW (BOTH PRACTICAL AND FUN!)

The truth is that you already are what you are seeking.

—ADYASHANTI

Having had squillions of conversations with women since pretty much forever, I have come across a few things that many women and PWPs don't know, but that all of them should be aware of. I could probably write an entire other book on this topic, but in this one I wanted to include just the answers and tips I think are likely to be most relevant to you. Like what to do about PMS and cramping, these are the answers that everyone should have in her toolbox.

When Can I Get Pregnant?

Most people have a vague idea that you can get pregnant between your periods, around the middle of the month. But they're not exactly sure, and maybe, well, maybe you can get pregnant anytime. "Is that right?" they often ask me, a little embarrassed that they actually don't know the answer—even the ones who've had babies! It's true that getting pregnant has everything to do with where you are in your cycle, but you have to understand what's happening inside you in order to be able to make the most effective use of timing.

Just to be sure, let's start at the beginning and do a little review.

Please note: This explanation is *not* intended to be a comprehensive natural family-planning course for you to use to prevent unwanted pregnancy! Rather, it's an overview to help empower you with some basic facts.

Many women think that the day of ovulation is the one and only day you can get pregnant. That's a serious bit of misinformation. There's actually a stretch of fertile time that lasts six days. This time frame includes the four days before ovulation—so, if you're having a twenty-eight-day cycle, cycle days 10 to 13—the day of ovulation, and the day after ovulation, you're fertile from about cycle day 10 to about cycle day 15.

Sounds easy, right? Just avoid sex on those days and you're free and clear—and not pregnant, right? Not quite, because there's one important caveat: sperm can live inside you for up to four days. So, to be really thorough, we need to extend the fertile window to include cycle days 6 to 16.

I know, that's a lot more than just one day, but knowing this will help you understand your exposure and modify your behavior appropriately.

In order to count the day correctly we need to start on the same day. We call that cycle day 1, which is the first day of bleeding. This day is important because it starts the counting by which you will predict the day you ovulate and the day you will begin your next period. If you have spotting, don't start the count until your first full day of bleeding.

An average cycle ranges between twenty-six and thirty-two days. Twenty-eight days is best, based on my clinical experience. It's important to track your cycle so you can know approximately how long it tends to be. Once you know that, you can predict when you're going to ovulate, which is the key factor when it comes to getting pregnant. You ovulate approximately fourteen days before your period begins. So, if you have a twenty-eight-day cycle, you'll ovulate around cycle day 14 (for some people, this can vary, but typically it's day 14). Once you have figured out the length of your cycle, do the math to adjust ahead or behind that date. Say you have a thirty-two-day cycle; you subtract fourteen from thirty-two to get your approximate ovulation date. That means you'll be ovulating on cycle day 18. That, in turn, means you should have sex on cycle days 13, 15, 17, and 19, if you want to get pregnant. If you have any doubt that you ovulated, throw in extra sex time on cycle day 21.

If you are trying to *avoid pregnancy*, remember you should use cycle tracking only as an adjunct tool (unless you are totally fine having an unplanned pregnancy) as there is a significantly larger margin of error with this method.

Just to clear up one last myth about ovulation: many folks believe that you cannot get pregnant while you're bleeding. Not true! Having your period means that you didn't get pregnant during the last cycle and your body is getting rid of the material that would have nurtured a developing baby so it can start fresh. But if you tend to have a short cycle (less than twenty-six days) and you're on cycle day 6 or 7 *and* you're still bleeding, it's possible that you might be ovulating early for the next cycle—which means you could get pregnant. So, getting pregnant while you're still bleeding may not be super common, but it is possible.

If I'm Trying to Conceive (TTC), Should I Use an Ovulation Detector Kit?

Pretty much every woman I know who is TTC is obsessed with using ovulation predictor kits. And friends, they are expensive! For some reason, many of us feel as though if we have just one more data point to help explain to us why we aren't getting pregnant, we might uncover the magical truth—that little factoid might give us some semblance of control at a time in our lives when we feel utterly powerless. I totally get that.

But this is not the time to lean on ovulation predictor tests. Save your money (or use it to buy menstrual supplies for the homeless women and PWPs in your area).

Ovulation kits test how much luteinizing hormone (LH) is in your urine. Your LH level surges twenty-four to forty-eight hours before you ovulate—it's what sparks the ovulation process. But your level can't tell you for sure if you really do ovulate after that surge—all the test measures is the surge itself. And if you don't have a regular cycle, it can be tricky to know when to use the kit (most do include multiple tests for this reason).

Here's what I recommend instead: use what you've learned in this book. Track your cycle on the Brazen app or another app.

Two things can help you see that you have in fact ovulated:

1. **Your temperatures are biphasic.** This means that they are in the 97s in the first fourteen days and the 98s in the second fourteen days.

2. **You see a drop in temperatures around cycle day 14** that correlates with your cervical discharge.

It is possible to ovulate without seeing these factors, but if you do observe them, they're very strong evidence that you have ovulated.

Once you figure out your general cycle, have sex five days before ovulation and every other day until after the sixteenth day, and you pretty much can't miss your window. In fact, you'll be actually giving yourself two swings at the plate by having intercourse twice before ovulation—so to speak—to cover all of your bases.

This is way cheaper than using an ovulation predictor kit. More important, this method takes the pressure off both you and your mate to spring into action based on whatever your ovulation predictor kit is telling you.

Now, if you have super-irregular cycles, you may need those kits to help you pinpoint any signs of ovulation. But otherwise, most folks don't need to use them.

Can I Get Cheap Biodegradable Home Pregnancy Tests?

Speaking of tests: how many home pregnancy tests have you taken in your life? Ten? Twenty? More? Then you know that the costs add up fast.

Home pregnancy tests are pretty cool because they can easily check the amount of human chorionic gonadotropin (hCG), aka the pregnancy hormone, in your urine. If you use them correctly, they're around 99 percent accurate and can tell you if you're pregnant quite early—from a day or two before when your period is due to a few days after you miss it and, of course, later on, too.

The downside? These guys typically cost around $20 apiece and are super bad for the environment. Each one is good for only one use, and they use a lot of nonrecyclable plastic.

Get ready for this: you can get super-cheap pregnancy tests without the plastic. You do have to pee into a little cup and dip the paper in, but to save almost $20, it's a no-brainer. You can find them on Amazon for practically pennies, which is a *way* better deal. As always, if your period doesn't come in the next week after a negative pregnancy test, you should consult with your doctor.

Here's how the tests work. When you're pregnant, your body starts producing hCG. This hormone is made right after a fertilized egg attaches to the wall of a woman's uterus. The hCG is concentrated in your urine, which makes it easy to test for. If hCG is present in the urine, it binds to proteins called antibodies and causes a color change in dye molecules on the test strip. On the pricey versions, this line appears only if the urine contains hCG—and hence the woman is pregnant. Sounds fancy and worth $20 a pop, right? Nope, not when you can buy the color-changing guts of the fancy kind for a fraction of the cost. It is super easy to read. Just as with the $20 ones, you will see either one or two lines. Two means you are having a baby.

Where Is My Clitoris?

In *Girls and Sex: Navigating the Complicated New Landscape,* a book that looked at the sexual attitudes and behaviors of college women, Peggy Orenstein reported that more than 70 percent of women don't know where their clitoris is located and, almost as bad, about 75 percent of all women never reach orgasm from intercourse alone—meaning without the extra help of sex toys, hands, or tongue. Is it a coincidence that about the same number can't find their own clitoris?

There are a *ton* of folks missing out on some serious bedroom delight. If you're one of them, hopefully this will help demystify the clitoris (aka "the clit") for you and give you access to some new avenues of pleasure.

The clitoris is a small, extremely sensitive organ that women have—apparently only to give them pleasure. It doesn't play the direct role in reproduction that the vagina and the penis do, but stimulating it can lead to orgasm, if done properly. There's a caveat only because there are so many nerve endings in the clitoris and it's so sensitive to touch that it can take a while to figure out just how best to touch it.

Of course, to do that, you have to know where it is! Every woman's vulva and clitoris look different. But the clitoris is mostly tucked inside a little hood inside the top of your inner labia, the "lips" that protect your sex organs. For some women, the tip of the clitoris will be clearly visible; for others, it may be pretty much hidden in its little hood. But either way, it reacts to touch, swelling and getting harder, much like the penis but apparently on a smaller scale—though, interestingly, it extends about five inches internally. (Which is actually pretty damn impressive.)

What to do if you aren't sure where your clitoris is? Check out this diagram, schedule some private time, put on some chill music, grab lots of lube (my anorgasmic patients report that CBD lube increases their ability to have an orgasm!), and just explore. You don't have to get anywhere, but do some gentle stroking around your external labia and vulva and see if you can find your clitoris. When you do, it is very likely to respond. Just remember, it's *super* sensitive—gentle touches will go a long way, especially at first.

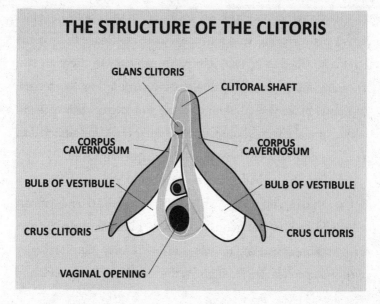

THE STRUCTURE OF THE CLITORIS

GLANS CLITORIS

CLITORAL SHAFT

CORPUS CAVERNOSUM

CORPUS CAVERNOSUM

BULB OF VESTIBULE

BULB OF VESTIBULE

CRUS CLITORIS

CRUS CLITORIS

VAGINAL OPENING

You can use this guide for your partners, too, if they need support in finding out your best places to be touched. Most important, have fun. Your body is yours to enjoy.

Is Masturbating Bad for Me?

Yikes. Talk about taboo. Hardly anyone wants to talk about this topic, but it's really important for women to have power in bed. Not necessarily power over their partners but power to enjoy themselves fully—by means of their own hands.

Whether or not they admit it (and chances are they don't publicly), a lot of people—no matter what their gender—masturbate. That means, just so we're all on the same page, that they touch their own sexual organs to bring themselves to orgasm, without a partner's help.

Even though it's extremely common, most people don't talk about masturbating, and for many, there continues to be some stigma attached to it. That may partly explain why there are still so many misconceptions about masturbation. For the record, it doesn't make you go blind or cause you to grow hair in weird places or make your sex organs swell up or leave you addicted so that you don't want to have sex with a partner anymore.

In fact, masturbating can be healthy for you in a number of ways. Orgasms, no matter what their cause, release endorphins, which make you feel good and reduce pain. Masturbating can ease tension, stress, and muscle pain and is *really good at relieving menstrual pain*. It also strengthens the muscles in your pelvic and anal area.

Equally important, masturbating helps you learn more about your body and what you like so that you can tell your sex partner(s) what really works best for you.[1] The payoffs are that, first, we can know how to please ourselves anytime we want, like a rock star, and second, we can share that knowledge with our partners.

Also, really important: if you masturbate, you're likely to be better able to identify any changes in your labia, vulva, clitoris, and anal area that could be pathological and get medical attention in a timely manner. Oftentimes your partners are distracted and might not pick up on such changes, plus I think it's always better not to delegate these kinds of responsibilities.

10

....

UNLEASHING OUR POWER

There are more than 2 billion people on this planet who menstruate. More than 80 percent of them are sick every single month with PMS, cramping or even *severe* cramping, nausea, extreme fatigue, PCOS, endometriosis (and don't forget, that can mean pain that is, say it with me: Worse. Than. A. Heart. Attack.), depression, fibroids, migraines, anemia, debilitatingly heavy flow, anxiety, bloating, acne, and more. Every month, women and PWPs lose anywhere from a few days to weeks of their lives to unnecessary suffering. Every day, girls miss school and the opportunity to learn because of menstrual cramps, which are the number one cause of school absenteeism in the United States.

Our society tells women and PWPs that all of this inconvenience and agony is normal—that suffering is simply part of being a woman and they should do it quietly because no one really wants to hear about their periods. It tells them that periods are too much of a hassle to deal with in drug and research studies, so everything will just be tested on men. It tells them that their cycles are gross and an embarrassing inconvenience for everyone else. It teaches them to be ashamed of a mechanism that allows our species to make humans out of almost nothing, starting with just one cell dividing into two. It monetizes this shame with products to sanitize and deodorize something that isn't dirty or malodorous, and then it taxes them for doing what we tell them to in order to make themselves acceptable to society. Too bad for the half billion women who, on any given day, don't have any supplies at all to manage their menstrual blood. Too bad they almost always miss school when they're sick and bleeding all over their clothes. But hey, that's normal.

Both women and men have internalized centuries-old myths, untruths, and damaging beliefs—that periods are filthy, that PWPs are filthy. That because of periods they—and let's be honest, we—are outcasts, inferior, less than. That because a crusty old white dude named Aristotle threw down some random thoughts about women more than two thousand years ago, we should all accept them as the definitive story of our normal bodily functions.

But the number one thing—the first thing—we need to do is simply not believe in those stories. Because *that's all they are*: stories. They are not truths, they are not even scientific or clinical facts. By understanding society's construction of periods as merely story, not truth, we can begin to disentangle ourselves from its hooks. As long as that story resonates with us as the truth in any way, we will be prisoners of its power and unable to change our present and future.

The sooner we recognize this, the sooner we can not only be freed from those stories but create some new, more badass ones that are a lot more true. The sooner we all collectively disembowel the old stories that have held us back, the sooner things will change.

The reality is that we cannot have a truly powerful women's movement, or women's anything, when 80 percent of us are sick every month. When women are experiencing epidemic levels of illness during menstruation and no one is talking about it. When no one is doing anything about our pain. When surgery and pharmaceuticals (which can play an important role in health care in other instances) are used to suppress and cut out our symptoms. Being sick and just having to deal with it or hide it is not a solution that will give us access to good health and power. It will never give us the resources to overcome our shame and stigma about menstruation and transmute it into authority and impact.[1]

In order to really prevail as PWPs, we have to reclaim our natural power. Our narrative about women being feeble, inferior, and weak is, as we know, total bullshit. We can push the equivalent of a turkey out of our vaginas, lose a significant amount of blood, and still get up the same night to nurse a baby three times. We experience pain as bad as heart attacks every single month and still show up at work with a smile on our face, even while we're silently crying inside, waiting for the day to end so we can go home and drink some wine and hope for the whole thing to just be over. We don't let anything get in our way.

One mom proved that there's more than one way to stop a car. As she was coming back with her shopping to her vehicle, her car started rolling toward a busy street with her twin girls in the back seat. She instinctively threw herself beneath the tires, thus slowing the vehicle and giving nearby neighbors enough time to run over and help stop the runaway car.[2] That's not feeble! Another mom was picking berries with her three-year-old daughter in Squamish, BC, when a cougar attacked, grabbing the little girl and rolling with her on the ground. She immediately wedged herself between the cougar and her child, stood up with the cat on her back, and "threw it off." No biggie. The little girl later asked, "Why didn't the kitty play nice?"[3] Women have superhuman powers, people!

But although we'll do almost anything for someone we love, we need to start doing something for ourselves. We need to stop apologizing for everything, staying quiet when we should scream, and adhering to society's stupid ideas about how we should look and feel about ourselves. In order to really move the needle in the world and embrace our true power, we need to start with our health. In order to have access to our deepest superhuman selves, we must toss out the old stories of shame, stigma, and filth and start to believe that we deserve good health and good periods. Because we do.

Telling a New Story

In my first career, I was a linguist. I studied cultural linguistics, a field that basically looks at how culture influences language and language influences culture. One important aspect of a culture is whether it's individualistic or collective—and its language will reflect and reveal this. The United States, Australia, Great Britain, Canada, the Netherlands, and New Zealand are all highly individualistic cultures that value hard work and ambition that benefits the individual person. Having those values means we become incredibly good at looking out for number one and allows us, as a culture, to innovate, create, and break down barriers set up by what people think is possible.

On the other hand, cultures in Asia, Africa, and South and Central America are more collectivistic in nature. They value putting the needs of the community ahead of the desires of individual people and promote selflessness. In those cultures, families and communities play a central role, and the society values doing what's best for the group overall.

These aren't just big ideas; they really impact our language and, as a consequence, our everyday behavior. A person from an individualistic culture will describe herself by saying "I'm a banker" or "I have a law degree" or "I'm a Gemini who loves swimming," while a person from a collectivistic culture might describe himself in terms of his relationships to other people, such as "I'm a good friend" or "I'm part of Habitat for Humanity."

One of my favorite words I came across in my previous career was the South African word *umbutu*, which means "I can experience my humanity only by experiencing your humanity." It's an amazing concept—and an empowering one. Guess what? Your health, and specifically your period health, impacts the lives of women everywhere.

You may be thinking "What in the hell is she talking about? How does my health impact anyone else's health (unless I have something contagious!), and more important, how does my period affect the lives of other women I don't even know?" I'll say it once more: *everything is connected*. My goal here is—as it has been throughout this book—to untangle the mind-set that we've had about our periods—and our health—until you see the interconnectedness of everything.

When we understand how every aspect of our bodies, our environment, and our cultures and societies at large are connected, only then can we really begin to figure out how to affect our world in a way that can create a sea of change and tell ourselves a new story about our periods, our bodies, our health, and our power.

But as you read this book, you were likely asking yourself "Okay, but how do I fix that? What can I do about that in relation to individual signs, symptoms, or issues?" These are important things to think about and part of the reason I wrote this book. I want you to feel better and have a normal period.

And (and this is a big *and*), remember that we're conditioned from birth to relate to our bodies, our environment, and our culture from a purely individualistic perspective. Approximately one-half of the people on the planet, including us in the United States, are part of an individualistic culture.

Why have I been talking about this difference between individualistic and collectivistic societies? Why is this an important distinction—and what does it have to do with our periods?

Since our society is individualistic, our cultural training has taught us to look at everything in isolation. So, we think of our symptoms just as our medical establishment does, taking one issue at a time and attempting to address just what's causing *that* symptom, as opposed to looking at the symptom as part of a whole system. That means we don't treat symptoms holistically—as part of what's going on in our body as a whole. And we definitely don't see them in relation to how society conceptualizes women.

When you think of your health, you'll likely fall into this type of individualistic thinking—which is totally okay, just realize that it's just not the whole picture. Just as we relate to each of our symptoms as a separate problem to be addressed on its own, we extrapolate that belief system and think that our general health is our own problem to fix.

It's true that in order to feel better, we need to take individual action, so that's a good thing. *But* (and this *but* is just as big as that *and*) as I mentioned before, the menstrual cycle—and let me be clear, I don't mean just *your* menstrual cycle but collectively *all* of our menstrual cycles—is in trouble. Around the planet, women are sick every single month from their cycles, and when they're sick, when they can't go to work, when they can't go to school, they can't create or contribute their genius. And when that happens, all of us PWPs suffer. The world suffers.

So yes, when we work on our own personal period health, we

can both improve our current situations *and* gain greater access to power and improved quality of life. And when we make the collective commitment to the health of all women as powerful as the commitment we have to ourselves, we can impact the experience of all women on the planet and potentiate their power and contributions as well as our own. And most important, *together* we can completely change the story.

The Story of Healthy Women

Healthy women break shit and make trouble. Remember when you were in elementary school and the PE teacher told the class that everyone was going to be playing kickball today? The teacher would usually assign the two best athletes or, worse, the two most popular kids to be the team captains. You know what came next: the systematic choosing of one child over another as the captains competed to build the most powerful, best-equipped teams for the Cyclones or the Tsunamis or whatever stupid names the PE teacher gave your teams.

Imagine if you were one of those team captains and 80 percent of the people you were choosing from were carrying hot-water bottles clutched to their abdomens. You might wonder, "Are those people the ones who are best equipped to win or not?"

Now imagine you had a group of strong, healthy women who looked ready and eager to start playing and go for the win. Sure, it might be harder to choose, but the game would be better— and more fun. We need stories where women don't need an automatic pass in PE when they have their periods. Where bleeding is as easy and painless as nodding. Where women—and men, for that matter—can walk into a drugstore and buy tampons without a hint of embarrassment. Where menstruating is a sign of power and contribution and women are proud of that demonstration. Where maybe men are even just a little bit jealous . . .

Right now, we don't even know what healthy women look like. And I don't mean look like as in "looks"—I mean, what would it actually look like in our world to have a bunch of healthy women running around?

Healthy women make trouble. Healthy women don't put up with shit. Healthy women fight back—for themselves, for their kids, for their planet. Healthy women don't put up with oppression. Healthy women don't buy lies; they change the story and tell the truth. Healthy women join together, assume control, and rule the world.

Vision for the Future

Pretty much all I do is talk to women from every walk of life who tell me that every month they're compromised and suffer from their periods. I can't help but think what would be possible if we helped women see that their periods don't have to feel like a curse; that, in fact, they're an instrument of unfair advantage. Our species cannot evolve without our cycles and our blood.

We have to educate women about their own bodies and cycles and do it in a way that teaches them dignity and self-respect for the contribution they're making possible.

My daughter recently started her period. She was telling me about her day and said, "Yeah, well, we went to dance, and then Spanish was a blow-off, and then I got my period . . ." (As if I wasn't going to notice that big news!) I was so excited and I hugged her so tightly (and cried a tiny tiny bit). She said, "Mom, I knew you were going to make a big deal out of this." I replied, "Of course I am. This is an amazing day. Today your body has made it clear that if you choose to, *you can make a human*! That is a privilege and pretty damn badass if you ask me. That means that you have just started to contact your deepest reserves of power, and I can't wait to watch the whole story unfold!" Then, to celebrate, I said, "Let's go out for a fancy dinner!"

She said, "Awesome. How about Chick-fil-A?" D'oh.

But it's not just women who have to move beyond the old stories. In addition to changing the language and attitudes we teach our girls, we have to do the same for young men. My cleaning lady, who is one of the most amazing humans ever, told me what she told her son before he went to middle school. I can't think of a better speech to give a twelve-year-old boy as he enters middle school. First, she talked to him about his changing body and what to expect on that front, but then she told him that girls' bodies were also starting to change in a way that would likely be very distracting to him. It was essential that he manage his reactions to the girls' bodies. That he should never comment or gawk, because that would be incredibly disrespectful and reveal that his character was weak. Then she said that the girls were going to get their periods. He asked what those were. Now, she's very religious, so her explanation has a religious slant, but you can see the general vibe of the message. She said, "Girls have something inside them called a uterus. That is the house in which the baby will grow. God puts really fresh healthy blood inside the uterus to make a really healthy place for the egg to implant and grow. But if a baby doesn't start grow-ing, the uterus can clean itself by eliminating that unused blood through the woman's vagina. And baby, when this happens, she will often suffer. She suffers for the fate of our species, and that is one of the most honorable things a human can do. So, when a girl has her period, you show her the deepest respect and kind-ness. Sometimes the blood will get on her clothes, and undigni-fied boys will tease her. If you see some blood on the back of a girl's jeans, you take off your jacket or sweatshirt and quietly hand it to her and tell her, 'You have a little something on the back of your jeans. You can give me my jacket back tomorrow.'"

By now I'm pretty sure you understand that you don't have to suffer, but I can imagine a world where boys are instructed to have deep respect and gratitude for our bodies and contribu-tion.

That's the sort of story I want to start hearing, telling, be-lieving. I imagine a world in which women are in sync with their periods, in which the information about our period health is used to exponentially decrease the risk of the diseases that kill us, such as cancer, diabetes, and heart disease (as well as suicide). I can imagine a time when women will be able to reclaim their self-esteem and self-worth by rejecting the previous centuries' old mythologies that are our real true curse. When women will be so connected to their health and power that they will be able to come together to support the uprising of all women on this planet. Once that happens, together we can transform our planet and the society that exists on it into something we can all feel proud of. I dream of a day in which my granddaughters, full of vitality and badassery, say to their friends, "Did you know that when my grandmother was young, women were really sick every month from their periods? Doctors said they were hysterical, treated them as if they had mental illness. It was so bad that many women even had their reproductive organs removed. It was so sad, they were so ashamed of their periods." And her friends will say, "No way, that's just a myth."

This is a very real possibility. We can change how we relate to the past—by intentionally speaking of it as it is: a story. We can change how we relate to our menstruating body by learning about what it is telling us and how to use that information to transform our health, cycles, fertility, future health, and the health of all other PWPs. We are more powerful than you can possibly imagine. That's why all of that mythology evolved—to control something men feared. It's time to reclaim our power, and in order to do so we need to start at the foundation: our health and cycles.

Now you can imagine. Imagine what your life would be if you felt great every day and your cycle was a blessing. Something invaluable and precious. And now imagine if that was how your daughter and sisters experienced their cycles and if your granddaughter never needed to hear this conversation because we were able to change the whole thing before she even set foot on this planet.

My friend Dan French is a comedian and once asked me what would happen if the women's movement won our battle. For a second, I didn't know what to say. No one had ever asked me before. When could we feel content and satisfied in our place in society? I said, "When everything is finally just equal." He laughed and said, "Are you serious? Dudes would never be satisfied with just getting things back to equal. We would be asking for retribution. At a minimum, for the last seventy years you couldn't vote. We would probably negotiate something like this: 'Considering the fact that we didn't get to vote for almost a century, we will be taking three votes for every one of your votes for the next thirty years and then see what we feel like doing.'"

Once again, I saw how easy it is for us, even when we are dreaming about what is possible, to be constrained by the conviction that we, as women, should be good girls and not ask for too much—even me, and I certainly don't identify myself as a good girl or rule follower. Still, when I had a world of possibility in front of me, I bunted with "equality."

What Liberation Looks Like

It's very simple. To be liberated would mean being free from the aspects of history that still stigmatize and shame us. We would be free to live in our bodies and our minds, and that living, in the end, would determine what we believe is possible and if we can achieve it.

My father told me more than a million times, "Everything

is possible until you allow your mind to make up a story to convince you otherwise."

I'd like to make up a new story today about what is possible for every woman and PWP on this planet. And I believe that what is possible when we change the story is actually beyond my grandest dreams. Won't you join me?

Acknowledgments

· · · · · · · · · ·

While this book took about nine months to write and publish, the content is the byproduct of twenty years of clinical experience and so many people along the way who helped me shape these ideas and theories and bring them to life. My co-founder, Witold (Rob) Krassowski, has been my partner in crime for the last ten years and without his genius, persistence, and ability to create order out of my chaos, I would never have been able to tell this story.

I also want to acknowledge my professor and mentor, Dr. Jaime Wu, who started the conversation that day in his office about how everything was related. It was that conversation that changed my life and my thinking forever.

Early on, my father, Paul Hurder, was my greatest influence. He convinced me that everything was possible and had I not believed that to be true, I would probably be in a wheelchair by now. And while my parents raised me when I was young, my adopted mom, Susan Susser, raised me to be the woman I am today. As a single mom, none of my work leading up to this book would have been attainable without her steadfast and unconditional support. She has made everything possible for me.

I have not had to look far for inspiration. My children, Wave and Ari, have helped me to stay focused, work from the heart, and even cook dinner on nights when I was writing and editing late into the evening.

Robert Schoenthaler, my partner and rock. You are the kindest and most loving person I have ever known. Thank you for being there every day and cheering me on throughout this process.

I want to thank Leslie Zieglar Schrock, my advisor at Brazen and friend, for introducing me to Simon and Schuster.

Many thanks to Jessica Branch for helping me pare down this book into something manageable and powerful, to Amiel Romain for your meticulous editing and feedback, and to Megan Neely for reading drafts and providing important content and conceptual feedback.

Thanks to my publisher Theresa DiMasi, editor Anja Schmidt, and the entire Tiller Press team for believing in the power of the period to change the lives and futures of all people with periods.

About the Author

· · · · · · · · · ·

Kirsten Karchmer is a CEO/founder/innovator in precision medicine and digital therapeutics, focusing on personalized nutraceuticals, lifestyle wellness, and biobehavioral interventions for women's health.

Kirsten is an integrative medicine practitioner and researcher with extensive experience in biomedical sciences, functional medicine, nutrition and digital health, mechanisms of mind-body healing, and evidence-based phytotherapies.

She has spent her entire adult career in the service of women's health and has helped more than ten thousand women over the last twenty years to improve their health, cycles, and fertility. In 2013, Kirsten translated her successful clinical programs into technology-enabled platforms that provide an affordable and scalable fertility solution. Her company Conceivable was named one of the most innovative health tech startups by MedTech in 2015, Best Fertility App by Healthline in 2016, and has been featured in TechCrunch, Fox News, *New York Observer*, PSFK, the Daily Dot, and Huffington Post.

Kirsten has presented at SXSW, Health 2.0, and Fertility Planit and lectures internationally on infertility, PCOS, endometriosis, women's health, the future of integrative medicine, and the use of technology to better serve patients, providers, and health care systems. Kirsten has been recognized as one of the top female startup founders to watch, is a recipient of the Texas Trailblazer Award for innovation in health care, and is a contributor to Huffington Post, mindbodygreen, and *Goop* magazine. Follow Kirsten on Facebook, Twitter, and LinkedIn.

Notes

Introduction

1. Sarah House, Thérèse Mahon, and Sue Cavill, "Menstrual Hygiene Matters: A Resource for Improving Menstrual Hygiene around the World," *Reproductive Health Matters* 21, no. 41 (2013): 257–59, https://www.tandfonline.com/doi/full/10.1016/S0968-8080%2813%2941712-3?scroll=top&needAccess=true.

2. Giovanni Grandi, Serena Ferrari, Anjeza Xholli et al., "Prevalence of Menstrual Pain in Young Women: What Is Dysmenorrhea?," *Journal of Pain Research* 5 (2012): 169–74, https://www.dovepress.com/prevalence-of-menstrual-pain-in-young-women-what-is-dysmenorrhea-peer-reviewed-article-JPR.

Chapter 1: What This Book Is About and Why It's Important

1. "Female Infertility," U.S. Department of Health & Human Services, Office of Population Affairs, February 21, 2019, https://www.hhs.gov/opa/reproductive-health/fact-sheets/female-infertility/index.html.

Chapter 2: The History of the Period: Nothing Has Changed for Menstruating Women in Centuries

1. Leviticus, in *The Holy Bible: Containing the Old and New Testaments: King James Version* (City: American Bible Society, 2010).

2. M.A.S. Abdel Haleem, translator, *The Qur'an: English Transla-*

tion and Parallel Arabic Text (New York: Oxford University Press, 2010).

3. Miyazaki Fumiko, "Female Pilgrims and Mt. Fuji: Changing Perspectives on the Exclusion of Women," *Monumenta Nipponica* 60, no. 3 (Autumn 2005): 339–91, https://www.jstor.org /stable/25066386?seq=1#page_scan_tab_contents.

4. Thomas Aquinas, "Question 92. The Production of the Woman," *The Summa Theologiæ of St. Thomas Aquinas*, New Advent, http://www.newadvent.org/summa/1092.htm.

5. Nicholas D. Smith, "Plato and Aristotle on the Nature of Women," *Journal of the History of Philosophy* 21, no. 4 (October 1983): 467–78, https://muse.jhu.edu/article/226997.

6. A. K. Gardner, "The Causes of Physical Degeneracy," *Popular Science Monthly* 1 (August 8, 1872): 482–91, https://en.wikisource .org/wiki/Popular_Science_Monthly/Volume_1/August _1872/The_Causes_of_Physical_Degeneracy.

7. Leviticus.

8. Petra Habiger, "Early History: Menstruation, Menstrual Hygiene and Woman's Health in Ancient Egypt," A Note from Germany, 1998, http://www.mum.org/germnt5.htm.

9. S. L. Read, "Thy Righteousness Is But a Menstrual Clout: Sanitary Practices and Prejudice in Early Modern England," *Early Modern Women: An Interdisciplinary Journal*, 3 (2008): 1–25, https://dspace .lboro.ac.uk/dspace-jspui/bitstream/2134/10271/2/READ -EMWJ2008v3.pdf.

10. Sabrina, "The History of the Sanitary Pad," Femme International, June 24, 2013, https://www.femmeinternational.org/the -history-of-the-sanitary-pad/.

11. Earle C. Haas, "US1964911A—Catamenial Device," July 3, 1934, Google Patents, https://patentimages.storage.googleapis.com/eb /bc/1c/3572a17ff720e9/US1964911.pdf.

12. "History of Tampax," Tampax, ///https://tampax.com/en-us /history-of-tampax.

13. J. A. Bryant, D. G. Heathcote, and V. R. Pickles, "The Search for 'Menotoxin,'" *The Lancet* 309, no. 8014 (April 2, 1977): 753, https://www.thelancet.com/journals/lancet/article/PIIS0140 -6736(77)92199-7/fulltext.

14. Kate Clancy, "Menstruation Is Just Blood and Tissue You Ended Up Not Using," *Scientific American*, September 9, 2011,

https://blogs.scientificamerican.com/context-and-variation
/menstruation-blood-and-tissue/?redirect=1.

15. Rahel R. Wasserfall, *Women and Water: Menstruation in Jewish Life and Law* (Hanover, NH: University Press of New England, 1999), https://bir.brandeis.edu/bitstream/handle/10192/32209 /Wasserfall.pdf?sequence=3&isAllowed=y.

16. Roni Caryn Rabin, "Free the Tampons," February 29, 2016, https://www.freethetampons.org/free-the-tampons.html.

17. Pliny the Elder, *Natural History: A Selection*, translated by John F. Healy (London: Penguin Classics, 1991); Janice Delaney, Mary Jane Lupton, and Emily Toth, *The Curse: A Cultural History of Menstruation* (Urbana: University of Illinois Press, 1988), 29–38.

18. A. K. Gardner, "The Causes of Physical Degeneracy," *Popular Science Monthly* 1 (August 8, 1872): 482–91, https://en.wikisource .org/wiki/Popular_Science_Monthly/Volume_1/August _1872/The_Causes_of_Physical_Degeneracy.

19. T. R. Sethna, *Vendidad: The Law of Zarathushtra to Turn Away from Evil* (Karachi: Sethna, 1977); Lebogang Keolebogile Maruapula, "Menstruation Myth: Why Are African Women Still Paying for It?," World Economic Forum, May 9, 2016, https://www .weforum.org/agenda/2016/05/menstruation-myth-why-are -african-women-still-paying-for-it/.

20. *Torah*, edited by Irmtraud Fischer and Mercedes Navarro Puerto (Atlanta: Society of Biblical Literature, 2014).

Chapter 3: Many Lies and a Truth:
Reframing the Language and Stigma Around Periods

1. "Top Euphemisms for 'Period' by Language," Clue, March 10, 2016, https://helloclue.com/articles/culture/top-euphemisms -for-period-by-language.

2. "National Population by Characteristics: 2010–2018," United States Census Bureau, https://www.census.gov/data/tables/time -series/demo/popest/2010s-national-detail.html.

3. Giovanni Grandi, Serena Ferrari, Anjeza Xholli et al., "Prevalence of Menstrual Pain in Young Women: What Is Dysmenorrhea?," *Journal of Pain Research* 5 (2012): 169–74, https://www .ncbi.nlm.nih.gov/pmc/articles/PMC3392715/.

4. Ibid.

5. Ashraf Direkvand-Moghadam, Kourosh Sayehmiri, Ali Delpisheh,

and Satar Kaikhavandi, "Epidemiology of Premenstrual Syndrome (PMS)—A Systematic Review and Meta-Analysis Study," *Journal of Clinical and Diagnostic Research* 8, no. 2 (February 2014): 106–9, https://pdfs.semanticscholar.org/0434/b5f746b26715c9d4 484901ca353d439accd2.pdf.

6. Jacqueline Thielen, "Premenstrual Dysphoric Disorder (PMDD): Different from PMS?," Mayo Clinic, November 29, 2018, https://www.mayoclinic.org/diseases-conditions/premenstrual-syndrome /expert-answers/pmdd/faq-20058315.

7. Direkvand-Moghadam et al., "Epidemiology of Premenstrual Syndrome (PMS)—A Systematic Review and Meta-Analysis Study."

8. Omur Taskin, Kiran Rikhraj, Justin Tan et al., "Link Between Endometriosis, Atherosclerotic Cardiovascular Disease, and the Health of Women Midlife," *The Journal of Minimally Invasive Gynecology* 26, no. 5 (July–August 2019): 781–84, https://www .jmig.org/article/S1553-4650(19)30206-7/abstract.

9. Fan Mu, Janet Rich-Edwards, Eric B. Rimm et al., "Association Between Endometriosis and Hypercholesterolemia or Hypertension," *Hypertension* 70, no. 1 (July 2017): 59–65, https://www .ahajournals.org/doi/full/10.1161/HYPERTENSIONAHA .117.09056.

10. George Miiro, Rwamahe Rutakumwa, Jessica Nakiyingi-Miiro et al., "Menstrual Health and School Absenteeism among Adolescent Girls in Uganda (MENISCUS): A Feasibility Study," *BMC Women's Health* 18, article no. 4 (January 3, 2018), https://bmcwomens health.biomedcentral.com/articles/10.1186/s12905-017-0502-z.

Chapter 4: How to Read Your Period

1. Galia Oron, Liran Hiersch, Shiran Rona et al., "Endometrial Thickness of Less than 7.5 mm Is Associated with Obstetric Complications in Fresh IVF Cycles: A Retrospective Cohort Study," *Reproductive BioMedicine Online* 37, no. 3 (September 2018): 341–48, https://www.rbmojournal.com/article/S1472-6483(18)30314-6 /abstract.

2. Rebecca Moffat, Sjanneke Beutler, Andreas Schötzau et al., "Endometrial Thickness Influences Neonatal Birth Weight in Pregnancies with Obstetric Complications Achieved After Fresh IVF–ICSI Cycles," *Archives of Gynecology and Obstetrics* 296,

no. 1 (July 2017): 115–22, https://link.springer.com/article/10.1007/s00404-017-4411-z.

3. Luc Johan Frans Rombauts, R. McMaster, Caroline Motteram, and Shavi Fernando, "Risk of Ectopic Pregnancy Is Linked to Endometrial Thickness in a Retrospective Cohort Study of 8120 Assisted Reproduction Technology Cycles," *Human Reproduction* 30, no. 12 (December 2015): 2846–52, https://www.ncbi.nlm.nih.gov/pubmed/26428211.

4. S. A. Winer and A. J. Rapkin, "Premenstrual Disorders: Prevalence, Etiology and Impact," *The Journal of Reproductive Medicine* 51, no. 4 (suppl.) (April 2006): 339–47, https://www.ncbi.nlm.nih.gov/pubmed/16734317.

5. Karolina Maliszewska, Mariola Bidzan, Małgorzata Świątkowska-Freund, and Krzysztof Preis, "Medical and Psychosocial Determinants of Risk of Postpartum Depression: A Cross-sectional Study," *Acta Neuropsychiatrica* 29, no. 6 (December 2017): 347–55, https://www.cambridge.org/core/journals/acta-neuropsychiatrica/article/medical-and-psychosocial-determinants-of-risk-of-postpartum-depression-a-crosssectional-study/EBB4708E044C36801C3F863F2C12AF11.

6. Lori M. Dickerson, Pamela J. Mazyck, and Melissa H. Hunter, "Premenstrual Syndrome," *American Family Physician* 67, no. 8 (April 15, 2003): 1743–52.

7. Julia Potter, Jean Bouyer, James Trussell, and Caroline Moreau, "Premenstrual Syndrome Prevalence and Fluctuation over Time: Results from a French Population–based Survey," *Journal of Women's Health* 18, no. 1 (January 2009): 31–39, https://www.ncbi.nlm.nih.gov/pmc/articles/PMC3196060/; JoAnn V. Pinkerton, Christine J. Guico-Pabia, and Hugh S. Taylor, "Menstrual Cycle–Related Exacerbation of Disease," *American Journal of Obstetrics & Gynecology* 202, no. 3 (March 2010): 221–31, https://www.ajog.org/article/S0002-9378(09)00854-0/abstract.

Chapter 5: How to Biohack Your Period, Part 1: Medicine and Technology

1. Holly Grigg-Spall, "Nine Major Myths about the Pill—from Cancer to Weight Gain," *The Guardian*, February 25, 2019, https://www.theguardian.com/society/2019/feb/25/nine-major-myths-about-the-pill-from-cancer-to-weight-gain.

2. Kimberly Daniels and Joyce C. Abma, "Current Contraceptive Status Among Women Aged 15–49: United States, 2015–2017," Data Brief no. 327, Centers for Disease Control and Prevention, December 2018, https://www.cdc.gov/nchs/data/databriefs/db327-h.pdf.

3. Rachel K. Jones, "Beyond Birth Control: The Overlooked Benefits of Oral Contraceptive Pills," Guttmacher Institute, November 2011, https://www.guttmacher.org/sites/default/files/report_pdf/beyond-birth-control.pdf.

4. Ibid.

5. Daniels and Abma, "Current Contraceptive Status Among Women Aged 15–49: United States, 2015–2017."

6. Grigg-Spall, "Nine Major Myths about the Pill."

7. David F. Archer, G. Kovalevsky, Susan A. Ballagh, and G. S. Grubb, "Effect on Ovarian Activity of a Continuous-Use Regimen of Oral Levonorgestrel/Ethinyl Estradiol," *Fertility and Sterility* 84 (suppl. 1) (September 2005): S24, https://www.fertstert.org/article/S0015-0282(05)01515-3/abstract; Paolo Vercellini, Giada Frontino, Olga De Giorgi et al., "Continuous Use of an Oral Contraceptive for Endometriosis-Associated Recurrent Dysmenorrhea That Does Not Respond to a Cyclic Pill Regimen," *Fertility and Sterility* 80, no. 3 (September 2003): 560–63, https://www.fertstert.org/article/S0015-0282(03)00794-5/fulltext; Alison Edelman, Robyn Lew, Carrie Cwiak, Mark Nichols et al., "Acceptability of Contraceptive-Induced Amenorrhea in a Racially Diverse Group of US Women," *Contraception* 75, no. 6 (June 2007): 450–53, https://www.contraceptionjournal.org/article/S0010-7824(07)00114-X/fulltext; Marcie B. Schneider, Martin Fisher, Stanford B. Friedman et al., "Menstrual and Premenstrual Issues in Female Military Cadets: A Unique Population with Significant Concerns," *Journal of Pediatric and Adolescent Gynecology* 12, no. 4 (November 1999): 195–201, https://www.ncbi.nlm.nih.gov/pubmed/10584223.

Chapter 6: How to Biohack Your Period, Part 2: Lifestyle Changes

1. Ann Williamson and A. M. Feyer, "Moderate Sleep Deprivation Produces Impairment in Cognitive and Motor Performance Equivalent to Legally Prescribed Levels of Alcohol Intoxication," *Occu-*

pational and Environmental Medicine 57, no. 10 (November 2000): 649–55, https://www.researchgate.net/publication/12338629_Moderate_sleep_deprivation_produces_impairment_in_cognitive_and_motor_performance_equivalent_to_legally_prescribed_levels_of_alcohol_intoxication.

2. Esra Tasali, Rachel Leproult, David A. Ehrmann, and Eve Van Cauter, "Slow-Wave Sleep and the Risk of Type 2 Diabetes in Humans," *Proceedings of the National Academy of Sciences of the United States of America* 105, no. 3 (January 22, 2008): 1044–49, https://www.ncbi.nlm.nih.gov/pmc/articles/PMC2242689/.

3. Kelly McGonigal, *The Upside of Stress: Why Stress Is Good for You, and How to Get Good at It* (New York: Avery, 2016).

4. Alia J. Crum, Peter Salovey, and Shawn Achor, "Rethinking Stress: The Role of Mindsets in Determining the Stress Response," *Journal of Personality and Social Psychology* 104, no. 4 (April 2013): 716–33, https://goodthinkinc.com/wp-content/uploads/CrumSaloveyAchor_RethinkingStress_JPSP2013.pdf.

5. Michael Boschmann, Jochen Steiniger, Uta Hille et al., "Water-Induced Thermogenesis," *The Journal of Clinical Endocrinology & Metabolism* 88, no. 12 (December 2003): 6015–19, https://academic.oup.com/jcem/article/88/12/6015/2661518.

6. Hsing-Yu Chen, Ben-Shian Huang, Yi-Hsuan Lin et al., "Identifying Chinese Herbal Medicine for Premenstrual Syndrome: Implications from a Nationwide Database," *BMC Complementary and Alternative Medicine* 14, no. 1 (June 2014): 206, https://bmccomplementalternmed.biomedcentral.com/articles/10.1186/1472-6882-14-206; Y. Masuda, S. Ohnuma, J. Sugawara et al., "Behavioral Effect of Herbal Glycoside in the Forced Swimming Test," *Methods and Findings in Experimental and Clinical Pharmacology* 24, no. 1 (January–February 2002): 19–21, https://www.ncbi.nlm.nih.gov/pubmed/11980383; Kazuo Yamada, and Shigenobu Kanba, "Effectiveness of *Kamishoyosan* for Premenstrual Dysphoric Disorder: Open-Labeled Pilot Study," *Psychiatry and Clinical Neurosciences* 61, no. 3 (June 2007): 323–25, https://onlinelibrary.wiley.com/doi/full/10.1111/j.1440-1819.2007.01649.x; Su Hee Jang, Dong Il Kim, and Min-Sun Choi, "Effects and Treatment Methods of Acupuncture and Herbal Medicine for Premenstrual Syndrome/Premenstrual Dysphoric Disorder: Systematic Review," *BMC Complementary and Alternative Medicine* 14, no. 11 (Janu-

ary 10, 2014), https://www.ncbi.nlm.nih.gov/pmc/articles/PMC3898234/.

7. "Mental Health and Social Relationships," Economic and Social Research Council, May 2013, https://esrc.ukri.org/news-events -and-publications/evidence-briefings/mental-health-and-social -relationships/.

Chapter 8: Diagnosis Doesn't Mean You're Doomed

1. American Board of Oriental Reproductive Medicine, https://aborm.org/.

2. Cheri D. Mah, Kenneth E. Mah, Eric J. Kezirian, and William C. Dement, "The Effects of Sleep Extension on the Athletic Performance of Collegiate Basketball Players," *Sleep* 34, no. 7 (July 2011): 943–50, https://www.researchgate.net/publication/51469186 _The_Effects_of_Sleep_Extension_on_the_Athletic_Performance _of_Collegiate_Basketball_Players.

3. Kirtida R. Tandel, "Sugar Substitutes: Health Controversy over Perceived Benefits," *Journal of Pharmacology and Pharmacother-apeutics* 2, no. 4 (October–December 2011): 236–43, https://www.ncbi.nlm.nih.gov/pmc/articles/PMC3198517/.

4. Rachel Ehrenberg, "Artificial Sweeteners May Tip Scales Toward Metabolic Problems," *Science News*, September 17, 2014, https://www.sciencenews.org/article/artificial-sweeteners-may-tip -scales-toward-metabolic-problems.

5. "The Truth About Aspartame Side Effects," Healthline, March 5, 2018, https://www.healthline.com/health/aspartame-side-effects.

6. Yasmin Mossavar-Rahmani, Victor Kamensky, JoAnn E. Manson et al., "Artificially Sweetened Beverages and Stroke, Coronary Heart Disease, and All-Cause Mortality in the Women's Health Initiative," *Stroke* 50, no. 3 (March 2019): 555–62, https://www.ahajournals.org/doi/full/10.1161/STROKEAHA.118.023100.

7. Patricia O. Chocano-Bedoya, JoAnn E. Manson, Susan E. Hankinson et al., "Dietary B Vitamin Intake and Incident Premenstrual Syndrome," *The American Journal of Clinical Nutrition* 93, no. 5 (May 2011): 1080–86, https://academic.oup.com/ajcn/article/93/5/1080/4597745.

8. Pedro-Antonio Regidor and Adolf Eduard Schindler, "Myoinositol as a Safe and Alternative Approach in the Treatment of Infertile PCOS Women: A German Observational Study," *International*

Journal of Endocrinology (January 2016): 1–5, https://www
.researchgate.net/publication/307852484_Myoinositol_as_a
_Safe_and_Alternative_Approach_in_the_Treatment_of
_Infertile_PCOS_Women_A_German_Observational_Study.

9. Maria Grazia Porpora, Roberto Brunelli, Graziella Costa et
    al., "A Promise in the Treatment of Endometriosis: An Ob-
    servational Cohort Study on Ovarian Endometrioma Reduc-
    tion by N-Acetylcysteine," *Evidence-Based Complementary and
    Alternative Medicine* (2013), https://www.researchgate.net
    /publication/237057797_A_Promise_in_the_Treatment_of
    _Endometriosis_An_Observational_Cohort_Study_on
    _Ovarian_Endometrioma_Reduction_by_N-Acetylcysteine.

10. Ming Chen, Hua Zhang, Jing Li, and Gui-Rong Dong, "Clinical
    Observation on Acupuncture Combined with Acupoint Sticking
    Therapy for Treatment of Dysmenorrhea Caused by Endome-
    triosis," *Zhongguo Zhen Jiu* [Chinese Acupuncture and Moxibus-
    tion] 30, no. 9 (September 2010): 725–28, https://www.ncbi
    .nlm.nih.gov/pubmed/20886791.

11. Andrew Flower, Jian Ping Liu, Sisi Chen et al., "Chinese Herbal
    Medicine for Endometriosis," Cochrane Database of Systematic
    Reviews, July 8, 2009, https://www.cochranelibrary.com/cdsr
    /doi/10.1002/14651858.CD006568.pub2/full.

12. Alexandra Miller, Hoa T. Vo, Liang Huo et al., "Estrogen Recep-
    tor Alpha (ESR-1) Associations with Psychological Traits in
    Women with PMDD and Controls," *Journal of Psychiatric Re-
    search* 44, no. 12 (February 2010): 788–94, https://www.ncbi
    .nlm.nih.gov/pmc/articles/PMC2948969/.

13. Katrina M. Wyatt, Paul W. Dimmock, Peter Jones, and P. M.
    Shaughn O'Brien, "Efficacy of Vitamin B-6 in the Treatment
    of Premenstrual Syndrome: Systematic Review," *BMJ Clini-
    cal Research* 318, no. 7195 (June 1999): 1375–81, https://
    www.researchgate.net/publication/12963484_Efficacy_of
    _vitamin_B-6_in_the_treatment_of_premenstrual_syndrome
    _Systematic_review.

14. Fabio Facchinetti, Paola Borella, Grazia Sances et al., "Oral Mag-
    nesium Successfully Relieves Premenstrual Mood Changes," *Ob-
    stetrics & Gynecology* 78, no. 2 (September 1991): 177, https://
    www.researchgate.net/publication/21087789_Oral_magnesium
    _successfully_relieves_premenstrual_mood_changes.

15. R. A. Sherwood, B. F. Rocks, A. Stewart, and R. S. Saxton, "Magnesium and the Premenstrual Syndrome," *Annals of Clinical Biochemistry* 23, no. 6 (November 1986): 667–70, https://journals.sagepub.com/doi/pdf/10.1177/000456328602300607.

16. Fotini Sampalis, Roxandra Bunea, Marie France Pelland et al., "Evaluation of the Effects of Neptune Krill Oil™ on the Management of Premenstrual Syndrome and Dysmenorrhea," *Alternative Medicine Review* 8, no. 2 (May 8, 2003): 171–79, https://pdfs.semanticscholar.org/2161/b69522192f570b0ae2ef179bf311fa5727e9.pdf.

17. M. Kathleen B. Lustyk, Winslow G. Gerrish, Haley Douglas et al., "Relationships Among Premenstrual Symptom Reports, Menstrual Attitudes, and Mindfulness," *Mindfulness* 2, no. 1 (March 2011): 37–48, https://www.ncbi.nlm.nih.gov/pmc/articles/PMC4859870/.

18. Karen Bluth, Susan Ann Gaylord, Khanh C. Nguyen et al., "Mindfulness-based Stress Reduction as a Promising Intervention for Amelioration of Premenstrual Dysphoric Disorder Symptoms," *Mindfulness* 6, no. 6 (December 2015): 1292–302, https://link.springer.com/article/10.1007%2Fs12671-015-0397-4.

19. "Quick Facts About Infertility," American Society for Reproductive Medicine, https://www.reproductivefacts.org/faqs/quick-facts-about-infertility/.

20. "Final CSR for 2016," Society for Assisted Reproductive Technology, 2019, https://www.sartcorsonline.com/rptCSR_PublicMultYear.aspx?ClinicPKID=0.

21. Ajani Chandra, Casey Copen, and Elizabeth Hervey Stephen, "Infertility and Impaired Fecundity in the United States, 1982–2010: Data from the National Survey of Family Growth," *National Health Statistics Reports* 67 (August 14, 2013): 1–18, https://www.ncbi.nlm.nih.gov/pubmed/24988820.

22. "Final CSR for 2016."

23. Mossavar-Rahmani et al., "Artificially Sweetened Beverages and Stroke, Coronary Heart Disease, and All-Cause Mortality in the Women's Health Initiative."

24. Thomas Brodin, Torbjörn Bergh, Lars Berglund et al., "Menstrual Cycle Length Is an Age-Independent Marker of Female Fertility: Results from 6271 Treatment Cycles of In Vitro Fertilization," *Fertility and Sterility* 90, no. 5 (November 2008): 1656–661,

https://www.fertstert.org/article/S0015-0282(07)03659-X
/fulltext.

25. Jerome H. Check, Harriet Adelson, Debbie Lurie, and Terri Jamison, "Effect of the Short Follicular Phase on Subsequent Conception," *Gynecologic and Obstetric Investigation* 34, no. 3 (1992): 180–83, https://www.ncbi.nlm.nih.gov/pubmed/1427421.

26. Jerome H. Check, Jordan Liss, Karen Shucoski, and Matthew L. Check, "Effect of Short Follicular Phase with Follicular Maturity on Conception Outcome," *Clinical and Experimental Obstetrics and Gynecology* 30, no. 4 (2003): 195–96, https://www.ncbi.nlm.nih.gov/pubmed/14664409.

27. Veronika Engert, Jonathan Smallwood, and Tania Singer, "Mind Your Thoughts: Associations Between Self-Generated Thoughts and Stress-Induced and Baseline Levels of Cortisol and Alpha-Amylase," *Biological Psychology* 103 (December 2014): 283–91, https://www.sciencedirect.com/science/article/pii/S030 1051114002191.

28. Lauren A. Wise, Kenneth J. Rothman, Ellen M. Mikkelsen, et al., "A Prospective Cohort Study of Physical Activity and Time to Pregnancy," *Fertility and Sterility* 97, no. 5 (May 2012): 1136–42, https://www.fertstert.org/article/S0015-0282(12)00259-2/fulltext.

29. Johanne Sundby and Berit Schei, "Infertility and Subfertility in Norwegian Women Aged 40–42: Prevalence and Risk Factors," *Acta Obstetricia et Gynecologica Scandinavica* 75, no. 9 (November 1996): 832–37, https://www.ncbi.nlm.nih.gov/pubmed /8931508.

30. Rakesh Sharma, Kelly R. Biedenharn, Jennifer M. Fedor, and Ashok Agarwal, "Lifestyle Factors and Reproductive Health: Taking Control of Your Fertility," *Reproductive Biology and Endocrinology* 11, no. 1 (July 16, 2013): 66, https://www.ncbi.nlm.nih.gov/pmc/articles/PMC3717046/.

31. Jorge Chavarro, Janet W. Rich-Edwards, Bernard A. Rosner, and Walter C. Willett, "A Prospective Study of Dietary Carbohydrate Quantity and Quality in Relation to Risk of Ovulatory Infertility," *European Journal of Clinical Nutrition* 63, no. 1 (October 2007): 78–86, https://www.researchgate.net /publication/5961249_A_prospective_study_of_dietary _carbohydrate_quantity_and_quality_in_relation_to_risk _of_ovulatory_infertility.

32. Jorge E. Chavarro, Janet W. Rich-Edwards, Bernard A. Rosner, and Walter C. Willett, "Dietary Fatty Acid Intakes and the Risk of Ovulatory Infertility," *American Journal of Clinical Nutrition* 85, no. 1 (January 2007): 231–37, https://www.ncbi.nlm.nih.gov /pubmed/17209201.

33. Jorge E. Chavarro, Janet W. Rich-Edwards, Bernard A. Rosner, and Walter C. Willett, "Protein Intake and Ovulatory Infertility," *American Journal of Obstetrics and Gynecology* 198, no. 2 (February 2008): 210, https://www.ajog.org/article/S0002-9378 (07)00833-2/abstract.

34. A. M. Clark, B. Thornley, L. Tomlinson, et al., "Weight Loss in Obese Infertile Women Results in Improvement in Reproductive Outcome for All Forms of Fertility Treatment," *Human Reproduction* 13, no. 6 (July 1998): 1502–5, https://www.researchgate .net/publication/13597592_Weight_loss_in_obese_infertile _women_results_in_improvement_in_reproductive_outcome _for_all_forms_of_fertility_treatment.

35. Chavarro et al., "A Prospective Study of Dietary Carbohydrate Quantity and Quality in Relation to Risk of Ovulatory Infertility."

36. Chavarro et al., "Dietary Fatty Acid Intakes and the Risk of Ovulatory Infertility."

37. Yuichi Ogino, Takahiro Kakeda, Koji Nakamura, and Shigeru Saito, "Dehydration Enhances Pain-Evoked Activation in the Human Brain Compared with Rehydration," *Anesthesia & Analgesia* 118, no. 6 (June 2014): 1317–25, https://journals.lww .com/anesthesia-analgesia/Fulltext/2014/06000/Dehydration _Enhances_Pain_Evoked_Activation_in_the.23.aspx.

38. Michael D. Curley and Robert N. Hawkins, "Cognitive Performance during a Heat Acclimatization Regimen," *Aviation, Space, and Environmental Medicine* 54, no. 8 (August 1983): 709–13, https://psycnet.apa.org/record/1983-32147-001; Kristen E. D'Anci, Caroline R. Mahoney, Arjun Vibhakar et al., "Voluntary Dehydration and Cognitive Performance in Trained College Athletes," *Perceptual and Motor Skills* 109, no. 1 (August 2009): 251–69, https://ase.tufts.edu/psychology/spacelab/pubs/DAnciEt AlHydrationPMS_2009.pdf.

39. D. F. Katz, D. A. Slade, and S. T. Nakajima, "Analysis of Preovulatory Changes in Cervical Mucus Hydration and Sperm Penetrability," *Advances in Contraception* 13, nos. 2–3 (June

1997): 143–51, https://link.springer.com/article/10.1023%2F
A%3A1006543719401.

40. Erato M. Stefanidou, Laura Caramellino, Ambra Patriarca, and
    Guido Menato, "Maternal Caffeine Consumption and *sine Causa*
    Recurrent Miscarriage," *European Journal of Obstetrics & Gynecol-
    ogy and Reproductive Biology* 158, no. 2 (October 2011): 220–24,
    https://www.ejog.org/article/S0301-2115(11)00240-5/abstract.

41. Sven Cnattingius, Lisa B. Signorello, Göran Annerén et al.,
    "Caffeine Intake and the Risk of First-Trimester Spontaneous
    Abortion," *The New England Journal of Medicine* 343, no. 25 (De-
    cember 21, 2000): 1839-45, https://pdfs.semanticscholar.org/7
    d92/4412519a3662beb6ffb483f1b907af2e4279.pdf.

42. Allen Wilcox, Clarice Weinberg, and Donna Baird, "Caffeinated
    Beverages and Decreased Fertility," *The Lancet* 332, no. 8626
    (December 31, 1988): 1453–56, https://www.ncbi.nlm.nih.gov
    /pubmed/2904572.

43. Ibid.

44. Rosemarie B. Hakim, Ronald H. Gray, and Howard Zacur, "Alco-
    hol and Caffeine Consumption and Decreased Fertility," *Fertil-
    ity and Sterility* 70, no. 4 (October 1998): 632–37, https://www
    .fertstert.org/article/S0015-0282(98)00257-X/fulltext.

45. Jan Gill, "The Effects of Moderate Alcohol Consumption on
    Female Hormone Levels and Reproductive Function," *Alcohol
    and Alcoholism* 35, no. 5 (September 2000): 417–23, https://
    academic.oup.com/alcalc/article/35/5/417/206575.

46. Gayle C. Windham, Laura Fenster, and Shanna H. Swan, "Mod-
    erate Maternal and Paternal Alcohol Consumption and the Risk
    of Spontaneous Abortion," *Epidemiology* 3, no. 4 (July 1992):
    364–70, https://www.ncbi.nlm.nih.gov/pubmed/1637900.

47. Rachel Leproult, Georges Copinschi, Orfeu Buxton, and Eve
    Van Cauter, "Sleep Loss Results in an Elevation of Cortisol Lev-
    els the Next Evening," *Sleep* 20, no. 10 (October 1977): 865–70,
    https://www.ncbi.nlm.nih.gov/pubmed/9415946.

48. Pablo A. Nepomnaschy, Kathy Welch, Dan McConnell et al.,
    "Stress and Female Reproductive Function: A Study of Daily
    Variations in Cortisol, Gonadotrophins, and Gonadal Steroids
    in a Rural Mayan Population," *American Journal of Human Biol-
    ogy* 16, no. 5 (September–October 2004): 523–32, https://www
    .ncbi.nlm.nih.gov/pubmed/15368600.

49. Karine Spiegel, Rachel Leproult, Mireille L'Hermite-Balériaux et al., "Leptin Levels Are Dependent on Sleep Duration: Relationships with Sympathovagal Balance, Carbohydrate Regulation, Cortisol, and Thyrotropin," *The Journal of Clinical Endocrinology & Metabolism* 89, no. 11 (November 2004): 5762–71, https://academic.oup.com/jcem/article/89/11/5762/2844744.

50. G. Anifandis, E. Koutselini, K. Louridas et al., "Estradiol and Leptin as Conditional Prognostic IVF Markers," *Reproduction* 129, no. 4 (April 2005): 531–34, https://rep.bioscientifica.com/view/journals/rep/129/4/1290531.xml?ck=nck.

51. J. D. Brannian, "Obesity and Fertility," *South Dakota Medicine* 67, no.7 (July2011):251–54,https://www.ncbi.nlm.nih.gov/pubmed/21848022; Ben Kroon, Keith Harrison, Nicole Martin et al., "Miscarriage Karyotype and Its Relationship with Maternal Body Mass Index, Age, and Mode of Conception," *Fertility and Sterility* 95, no. 5 (April 2011): 1827–29, https://www.fertstert.org/article/S0015-0282(10)02924-9/fulltext.

52. M.A.Q. Mutsaerts, H. Groen, H. G. Huiting et al., "The Influence of Maternal and Paternal Factors on Time to Pregnancy—A Dutch Population-Based Birth-Cohort Study: The GECKO Drenthe Study," *Human Reproduction* 27, no. 2 (February 2012): 583–93, https://academic.oup.com/humrep/article/27/2/583/2919339.

53. A. M. Clark, B. Thornley, L. Tomlinson, et al., "Weight Loss in Obese Infertile Women Results in Improvement in Reproductive Outcome for All Forms of Fertility Treatment," *Human Reproduction* 13, no. 6 (July 1998): 1502–5, https://www.researchgate.net/publication/13597592_Weight_loss_in_obese_infertile_women_results_in_improvement_in_reproductive_outcome_for_all_forms_of_fertility_treatment.

54. Ibid.

55. S. L. Gudmundsdottir, W. D. Flanders, and L. B. Augestad, "Physical Activity and Fertility in Women: The North-Trøndelag Health Study," *Human Reproduction* 24, no. 12 (December 2009): 3196–204, https://academic.oup.com/humrep/article/24/12/3196/647657.

56. Ibid.

57. Karin Ried, "Chinese Herbal Medicine for Female Infertility: An

Updated Meta-analysis," *Complementary Therapies in Medicine* 23, no. 1 (February 2015): 116–28, https://www.sciencedirect.com/science/article/pii/S0965229914001915?via%3Dihub.

58. Li Tan, Yao Tong, Stephen Cho Wing Sze, et al., "Chinese Herbal Medicine for Infertility with Anovulation: A Systematic Review," *The Journal of Alternative and Complementary Medicine* 18, no. 12 (November 30, 2012): 1087–100, https://www.liebertpub.com/doi/abs/10.1089/acm.2011.0371?rfr_dat=cr_pub%3Dpubmed&url_ver=Z39.88-2003&rfr_id=ori%3Arid%3Acrossreforg&journalCode=acm.

59. A. Galhardo, J. Pinto-Gouveia, M. Cunha, and M. Matos, "The Impact of Shame and Self-Judgment on Psychopathology in Infertile Patients," *Human Reproduction* 26, no. 9 (September 2011): 2408–14, https://academic.oup.com/humrep/article/26/9/2408/724311.

60. Germaine M. Buck Louis, Kirsten J. Lum, Rajeshwari Sundaram et al., "Stress Reduces Conception Probabilities Across the Fertile Window: Evidence in Support of Relaxation," *Fertility and Sterility* 95, no. 7 (June 2011): 2184–89, https://www.fertstert.org/article/S0015-0282(10)01031-9/fulltext.

61. Wilcox, Weinberg, and Baird, "Caffeinated Beverages and Decreased Fertility."

62. C. D. Lynch, R. Sundaram, J. M. Maisog et al., "Preconception Stress Increases the Risk of Infertility: Results from a Couple-Based Prospective Cohort Study—The LIFE Study," *Human Reproduction* 29, no. 5 (May 2014): 1067–75, https://academic.oup.com/humrep/article/29/5/1067/2913997.

63. Richard Bränström, Pia Kvillemo, and Torbjörn Åkerstedt, "Effects of Mindfulness Training on Levels of Cortisol in Cancer Patients," *Psychosomatics* 54, no. 2 (March–April 2013): 158–64, https://www.sciencedirect.com/science/article/abs/pii/S003331821200076X?via%3Dihub.

64. Ibid.

65. Gill, "The Effects of Moderate Alcohol Consumption on Female Hormone Levels and Reproductive Function."

66. Galhardo et al., "The Impact of Shame and Self-Judgment on Psychopathology in Infertile Patients."

67. Heidi D. Nelson, Elizabeth Haney, Linda Humphrey et al., "Management of Menopause-Related Symptoms," *AHRQ Evidence*

Reports (Rockville, MD: Agency for Healthcare Research and Quality, 2005), https://www.ncbi.nlm.nih.gov/books/NBK37757/.

68. Maryam Mehrpooya, Soghra Rabiee, Amir Larki-Harchegani et al., "A Comparative Study on the Effect of 'Black Cohosh' and 'Evening Primrose Oil' on Menopausal Hot Flashes," *Journal of Education and Health Promotion* 7 (2018): 36, http://www.jehp.net/article.asp?issn=2277-9531;year=2018;volume=7;issue=1;spage=36;epage=36;aulast=Mehrpooya.

69. Mahmoud Rafieian-Kopaei and Mino Movahedi, "Systematic Review of Premenstrual, Postmenstrual and Infertility Disorders of Vitex Agnus Castus," *Electronic Physician* 9, no. 1 (January 2017): 3685–89, https://www.ncbi.nlm.nih.gov/pmc/articles/PMC5308513/.

70. Ibid.

71. Chang Ho Lee and Jong-Hoon Kim, "A Review on the Medicinal Potentials of Ginseng and Ginsenosides on Cardiovascular Diseases," *Journal of Ginseng Research* 38, no. 3 (July 2014): 161–66, https://www.sciencedirect.com/science/article/pii/S1226845314000499?via%3Dihub.

72. Soheila Ehsanpour, Kobra Salehi, Behzad Zolfaghari, and Soheila Bakhtiari, "The Effects of Red Clover on Quality of Life in Postmenopausal Women," *Iranian Journal of Nursing and Midwifery Research* 17, no. 1 (January–February, 2012): 34–40, https://www.ncbi.nlm.nih.gov/pmc/articles/PMC3590693/.

73. Barbara Grube, A. Walper, and Donna Wheatley, "St. John's Wort Extract: Efficacy for Menopausal Symptoms of Psychological Origin," *Advances in Therapy* 16, no. 4 (July–August 1999): 177–86, https://www.ncbi.nlm.nih.gov/pubmed/10623319.

74. Henry O. Meissner, Przemysław Michał Mrozikiewicz, Teresa Bobkiewicz-Kozłowska, et al., "Hormone-Balancing Effect of Pre-Gelatinized Organic Maca (*Lepidium Peruvianum Chacon*): (I) Biochemical and Pharmacodynamic Study on Maca using Clinical Laboratory Model on Ovariectomized Rats," *International Journal of Biomedical Science* 2, no. 3 (September 2006): 260–72, https://www.researchgate.net/publication/236894512_Hormone-Balancing_Effect_of_Pre-Gelatinized_Organic_Maca_Lepidium_peruvianum_Chacon_I_Biochemical_and_Pharmacodynamic_Study_on

_Maca_using_Clinical_Laboratory_Model_on_Ovariectomized
_Rats.

75. Rachael Link, "Best Omega-6 Foods, Surprising Benefits & Proper Ratio with Omega-3s," Dr. Axe, November 29, 2018, https://draxe.com/omega-6/.

76. Ibid.

77. S. Ziaei, A. Kazemnejad, and M. Zareai, "The Effect of Vitamin E on Hot Flashes in Menopausal Women," *Gynecologic and Obstetric Investigation* 64, no. 4 (2007): 204–7, https://www.ncbi.nlm.nih.gov/pubmed/17664882.

78. Nuray Cetisli, A. Saruhan, and B. Kivcak, "The Effects of Flaxseed on Menopausal Symptoms and Quality of Life," *Holistic Nursing Practice* 29, no. 3 (May 2015): 151–57, https://www.ncbi.nlm.nih.gov/pubmed/25882265.

Chapter 9: Before I Go, a Few Very Important Things Every Woman Should Know (Both Practical and Fun!)

1. "Where Is My Clitoris? Do I Even Have One?," Planned Parenthood, https://www.plannedparenthood.org/learn/teens/ask-experts/where-is-my-clitoris-do-i-even-have-one.

Chapter 10: Unleashing Our Power

1. Roni Caryn Rabin, "The Drug-Dose Gender Gap," *New York Times*, January 28, 2013, https://well.blogs.nytimes.com/2013/01/28/the-drug-dose-gender-gap/.

2. Lori Grisham, "Mass. Mom Saves Kids by Throwing Herself in Front of Car," *USA Today*, March 19, 2014, https://www.usatoday.com/story/news/nation-now/2014/03/19/massachusetts-mom-speedbump-saves-kids/6612509/.

3. Cathryn Atkinson, " 'Now She Knows What a Cougar Is,' " *The Globe and Mail* (British Columbia), May 2, 2018, https://www.theglobeandmail.com/news/british-columbia/now-she-knows-what-a-cougar-is/article4276779/.

Index